the HOLISTIC GUT PRESCRIPTION

the
HOLISTIC GUT
PRESCRIPTION

Create Your Own Personal Path
to Optimal Digestive Wellness

Lauren Deville, NMD

NEW YORK

LONDON • NASHVILLE • MELBOURNE • VANCOUVER

the HOLISTIC GUT PRESCRIPTION
Create Your Own Personal Path to Optimal Digestive Wellness

Published in New York, New York, by Morgan James Publishing. Morgan James is a trademark of Morgan James, LLC. www.MorganJamesPublishing.com

The Morgan James Speakers Group can bring authors to your live event. For more information or to book an event visit The Morgan James Speakers Group at www.TheMorganJamesSpeakersGroup.com.

ISBN 978-1-68350-667-6 paperback
ISBN 978-1-68350-668-3 eBook
Library of Congress Control Number: 2017910956

Cover Design by:
Rachel Lopez
www.r2cdesign.com

Interior Design by:
Bonnie Bushman
The Whole Caboodle Graphic Design

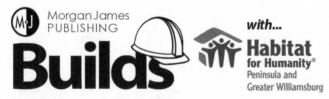

In an effort to support local communities, raise awareness and funds, Morgan James Publishing donates a percentage of all book sales for the life of each book to Habitat for Humanity Peninsula and Greater Williamsburg.

Get involved today! Visit
www.MorganJamesBuilds.com

TABLE OF CONTENTS

INTRODUCTION

I couldn't even remember what "normal" felt like.

As a child, I had severe allergies, in the usual pattern, called the "atopic triad": eczema and hives, then hay fever, then asthma. When I was little, I loved dresses and frills and everything sparkly, but my rashes were so severe that I'd claw my legs open at night until they bled. My mom dressed me in long pants to hide the carnage and keep me from continuing to scratch whenever possible. (She tells me now that I pouted about it a lot.)

I was born and spent the first few years of my life in Louisiana, but after multiple asthma attacks despite allergy shots, the allergist there told my family that perhaps I might do better in a drier climate. So, despite the fact that both my parents had lived in Louisiana for the better part of their lives, and all of my extended family was there too, my dad flew out to Arizona to look for a job—the driest of the dry states.

In short order, we moved. And it worked: I definitely improved. Over the years, I even appeared to "outgrow" my allergies (provided I wasn't around animals). As a physician myself now, though, I know that allergies are cumulative. The body reacts to environmental allergies, to food, and to chemicals in the same way: with histamine release. We succeeded in eliminating at least the environmental allergens in Louisiana, which knocked down my overall allergen load low enough that many of my symptoms faded to background noise… for a time. I don't know if I had chemical sensitivities back then, but in retrospect, I did have food allergies: the IgG kind, the kind you can't diagnose with a skin prick test (more on this in Chapter 1). Those symptoms don't go away if you don't address them—but I suspect that, with the strong healthy adrenals of a happy child, and the removal of the environmental allergens, my body was able to handle the food allergies without giving me too much trouble.

Yet.

My adrenals, the glands that help deal with stress (more on this in Chapter 4), took a major hit when my father died. I was fifteen. I suspect that they suddenly couldn't produce enough cortisol (the stress hormone, and also the anti-inflammatory hormone) to deal with a *normal* day, let alone inflammatory insults like the food allergies that had been there all along. It was shortly after that when I first got acne: before that, people used to tell me I had skin "like a porcelain doll." I think that was when the bloating began, too. Atopic children (those with the triad of skin problems, allergies, and asthma) commonly grow up to develop gut problems. I'd always had issues with constipation, but by the time I recognized the bloating for what it was, I was so used to it that I'd basically just tuned it out. I assumed everyone must feel this way.

Then in college, I must have been exposed to toxic mold. (I deduced this via bloodwork in retrospect—and I did live in some pretty questionable places in college.) I think college was when the eczema came back, too. If I didn't have leaky gut syndrome before (see Chapter 1), I had it now: and with it, overgrowth of candida (see Chapter 3), a fungal organism that eats sugar and simple carbohydrates and makes carbon dioxide as a byproduct.

And guess what I was eating? Simple carbs. *All* the *time.*

I thought I was being healthy, though: I ate bagels and cream cheese for breakfast, single-serve containers of fruited yogurt on the go, and occasionally I had iced mochas for lunch. (Okay, more than occasionally. The coffee cart guy gave me free coffee on a regular basis, and brought his wife to see me perform in a musical once.) But sometimes I'd snack on pieces of fruit here and there, maybe even the occasional carrots. I didn't really cook (it seemed I always had better things to do), but I wasn't eating fast food or desserts at every meal either, so I was doing well, right? I couldn't explain the fact that I felt several months pregnant every time I ate, but I didn't really think about it that much, to be honest. I was just so *used* to it.

As you might imagine, naturopathic medical school was a *bit* of a rude awakening.

I remember when I had my first food allergy test in the student clinic. The older student who took my case came back into the room with a somber look on her face. A sense of utter dread crashed over me.

"Please," I begged, "please, just tell me I'm not allergic to coffee!"

"No," she said, sliding the results over to me, "but you're allergic to everything else."

It was almost true. To date, I think I've only seen one or two other patient food allergy tests to rival my own.

Since then, it's been quite a journey. I cut out the foods I was sensitive to and then added them back six weeks later, but (unlike most patients) the sensitivities just returned. While the bloating improved, during school, it really never went away. I'm sure this had something to do with the fact that, as a medical student, I was a stress ball. I already had a predisposition to anxiety ("I have to do this, and this, and this, and oh my gosh, what if I forget that?"). I was in constant "fight or flight" mode—which meant all the blood flowed to my limbs, and not to my gut, where it should have gone to "rest and digest." I ate standing up, in the car, rushing to the next clinic rotation… anything but sitting down and chewing slowly, like I should have. This meant I wasn't releasing sufficient digestive enzymes to break down the food I'd just thrust into my gullet—so the bacteria in my gut happily did it for me, producing an abundance of carbon dioxide and acid byproducts in the process. The bloating and cramping became especially bad, I noticed, when I was on rotation with a few attending physicians who were… let's just say, not very nice to us students. (You know those stereotypes of medical school, where the attending physicians pick various students to humiliate at every opportunity? Yeah, that happens in naturopathic school, too. I never knew when it would be my turn to suffer wrath for something as simple as offering a patient a glass of water.) That entire quarter, and especially on one particular shift, I was one big gas bubble.

Meanwhile, the eczema waxed and waned, mostly in response to various homeopathic remedies, which I plied upon myself like a mad scientist, lacking the patience to submit myself to a student clinician with more experience and objectivity. Once, my arms exploded in rashes from shoulders to wrists. I looked like I'd been burned: I wore long sleeves for three weeks in the Arizona summer to cover them up. The acne also stubbornly refused to budge, though it was decidedly worse around my menstrual cycle. As a woman who cared about my appearance, that was almost worse than anything else.

Over those next four years of school, I tried a lot of things: a lot of diets, a lot of supplements, a lot of homeopathic remedies. My healthy regimen was enough to get me by, and make great strides, but not enough to get me fully better. My obstacles to cure were certainly stress (Chapter 5) and toxic thoughts—("There's never enough time and what if I don't get it all done?!"—see Chapter 7), but also mold and recurrent candida (see Chapters 3 and 4), which prevented the leaky gut (see Chapter 1) from fully healing. Because of the mold, I wasn't detoxing my hormones as well as I should have been either—which made everything worse around my cycle (see Chapter 6).

Each of my issues had to be addressed, fully, in order for my own gut to heal: leaky gut syndrome and food allergies, candida, mold, seasonal allergies, adrenal fatigue, histamine intolerance, hormone imbalance, anxiety and stress. Some of those symptoms stemmed from the same root cause, and some were a root cause in and of themselves. Combined, they created my specific brand of digestive dysfunction. Every case is a little bit different—that's why this is the *Holistic* Gut Prescription!

This book is divided into two main sections: Part One discusses common obstacles to a healthy gut, including all those I had to address myself, plus some other common ones that I frequently see in many of the patients who arrive at my clinic. These chapters will contain more information than many of you need, and not enough for others. Some chapters may not be important for your particular case at all; they are here because they represent a significant percentage of the root cause of gut dysfunction I see in my patient population. In order to determine which chapters are most important for you, I recommend that you take the following quiz to determine your customized road map through this book.

Which Are Your Most Likely Obstacles to Cure?

1. Do you have rashes or eczema? Y/N
2. Do you have GERD or reflux? Y/N
3. Do you have gas and bloating? Y/N
4. Do you have alternating constipation and diarrhea, or either one predominately? Y/N
5. Do you have any chemical sensitivities—i.e. problems walking down the cleaning aisle, dislike of perfumes or artificial scents? Y/N
6. Have you ever moved into a brand new home, or done any renovation in your home? Y/N
7. Have you ever lived or worked in a place you suspected to be moldy? Y/N
8. Do you have recurrent sinus infections? Y/N
9. Do you consider yourself to be a Type A personality, always taking on more tasks? Y/N
10. Do your symptoms follow a periodic, cyclical pattern, waxing and waning every few weeks? Y/N
11. Do you sometimes feel like you look pregnant after a meal? Y/N
12. Do you feel like there is a lot of stress in your life? Y/N
13. Did you develop symptoms suddenly after an acutely stressful event in your life? Y/N
14. a. If you are a woman, do you have trouble with your female hormones (PMS or perimenopausal symptoms)?
    b. If you are a man, do you suspect your testosterone might be low (fatigue, low motivation, depression, weight gain)? Y/N

15. Do you feel fatigued, and/or struggle with dry skin, weight gain, hair loss, or constipation? Y/N

16. Do you often feel hopeless? Y/N

17. Do you struggle with following through on your good health resolutions? Y/N

Key:

If yes to questions 1-4: Read Chapter 1

If yes to questions 5-6: Read Chapter 2

If yes to questions 7, 8, 10: Read Chapter 3

If yes to questions, 3, 4, 11: Read Chapter 4

If yes to questions 9, 12, 13: Read Chapter 5

If yes to questions 14, 15: Read Chapter 6

If yes to questions 16, 17: Read Chapter 7

Each chapter includes a summary at the end, called the Take-Home Message, of steps you can take *right now* to improve your digestive health. This summary encompasses the most important takeaways from each chapter. If you follow just those and ignore the rest, you will still likely see significant improvement. I will intersperse patient stories to help illustrate the concepts, as well. Names and identifying information have all been changed, of course. And fair warning: I believe the Bible has a lot of wisdom for addressing the mental and spiritual struggles that often comprise our primary obstacles to cure. (It's certainly made all the difference for me!) So in those chapters, I reference scripture often. If that doesn't resonate with you, feel free to skim or skip those chapters—or read them anyway, and keep what works for you.

Part Two will address how to *stay* better once you *get* better; and remember, the gut is not isolated! You can't maintain a healthy gut without maintaining a healthy body overall. Neglect any one of the building blocks for health presented here, and your issues are likely to recur. Many times, a patient will get healthy, and leave my clinic thrilled, only to come back a few months or years later with all the old symptoms back. When I ask what happened, the answer is always some variation on, "Well, once I got better, I went back to my old patterns, and it was okay for awhile, but then it caught up with me..."

This is the beauty of the naturopathic philosophy: our bodies are designed to heal themselves. If you give your body what it needs to heal and remove the obstacles to cure, health will generally follow. How simple or how complicated the interpretation of this principle becomes in a given case depends on a couple of main variables:

1. How many obstacles to cure are present,
2. How many building blocks are missing,
3. How long you've been in the present condition, and/or
4. How willing you are to make the necessary changes.

I'm assuming, if you've picked up this book, that you're willing! So we've got that one going for us.

I'm grateful you've decided to go on this journey with me, and look forward to helping you achieve the healthy digestion you've always wanted!

In Health,

Dr Lauren

Part 1

OBSTACLES TO A HEALTHY GUT

All of the various components of digestion have to work together in order for assimilation of nutrients to happen. Before we get into the obstacles, let's take a brief look at how things are *supposed* to work.

Digestion In A Nutshell (A.K.A. Bowel Transit)

When you chew your food, the enzymes in your saliva begin to break down the simple carbohydrates you consume, turning them into glucose. You swallow, and the food travels from your throat (A.K.A. *pharynx*) to your esophagus.

The function of your esophagus is to connect your throat to your stomach, but it's also a muscle, pushing your food downward in rhythmic waves called *peristalsis*.

The esophagus opens into the stomach via a small muscle called the esophageal sphincter. The sphincter is coordinated with the peristaltic waves, opening in response to the waves, and closing in response to the low pH of the stomach acid below it.

Your stomach processes the food bolus you've just swallowed, and produces hydrochloric acid which breaks down your food into bits for the next stages of the digestive process. Hydrochloric acid is especially necessary for breaking down protein; if there is too little, the later stages of digestion won't be able to assimilate nutrients that are still trapped in their organic material, leading to malabsorption. Also, if those bits of food can't go through later stages of digestion, the bacteria in your intestines will break it down for you, leading to gas and bloating.

Your stomach is also the place where you secrete Intrinsic Factor, a protein necessary for the later absorption of Vitamin B12.

Your stomach dumps food into your small intestine, where peristalsis continues. Your gut can only absorb simple molecules, so the first part of your small intestine, called the duodenum, receives digestive enzymes from the pancreas to further break down protein, carbs, and fat. Think of enzymes like pairs of scissors that cut bigger molecules into smaller pieces. There's a different pair of scissors, or different enzymes, for different types of food.

The duodenum also receives bile from your gall bladder (or directly from your liver if your gall bladder has been removed) to emulsify fat and allow its absorption. Bile works on fat the way soap works on dirt. Most toxins from solvents are fat-soluble, so if these have entered your digestive tract, the bile will sweep these up too.

Nutrients absorbed by the small intestine travel to the liver for processing. This is where your body packages triglycerides into cholesterol, and the main site of storage for certain nutrients like Vitamin A and iron. Any chemicals your intestines absorb that your liver doesn't recognize end up going through the liver's phases of detoxification at this stage as well, so that they don't circulate throughout your bloodstream. The liver is also the site of bile production; the gallbladder just stores it and secretes it into the intestines.

Beneficial bacteria, or probiotics, gobble up whatever's still not simple enough for your body to absorb, and they leave behind lactic acid as a byproduct. This process is called fermentation. A little chemistry digression here: fermentation happens in the absence of oxygen, and it's the conversion of carbohydrates (sugar) to alcohol or lactic acid, and carbon dioxide (CO_2). Lactic acid and/or alcohol act as a natural preservative, because bad bacteria cannot survive in an acidic environment—they keep the "bad" bacteria and yeast in check. They also break down antinutrients (called phytobiotics) that block the body's ability to absorb vitamins and minerals.

Actual absorption of nutrients occurs mostly in the second and third part of the small intestine, called the jejunum and the ileum. The ileum is also the site of absorption of Intrinsic Factor, which is bound to Vitamin B12.

After extracting all the good stuff, the ileum, the last part of the small intestine, then dumps whatever's left over into the colon. The colon consists of the cecum (the connection between the ileum and the rest of the colon), and then the ascending, transverse, and descending colon, which are what they sound like. The descending colon turns into the sigmoid colon, so named because it's shaped like an S, and it empties into the rectum. Peristalsis continues throughout the colon, pushing waste downward for elimination. The colon also reabsorbs water from the stool, so that it is neither too watery nor too dry.

The rectum is about eight inches long, and acts as a storage reservoir for stool. When it becomes full, the brain tells you that it's time to have a bowel movement (or to release gas, left over from the fermentation process above). The rectum is connected to the anal sphincter, part of the muscles of the pelvic floor. These are voluntary muscles that relax when we get to a toilet.

Ideally this whole process takes about 24 hours. For the rest of Part One, we'll look at reasons why things don't always happen this way.

Keep in mind as you read that the above "nutshell" is simplified. The body is composed of organs that are highly interrelated. For example, the gut also houses about 70% of your immune system; it's also where almost 90% of your serotonin (the feel-good neurotransmitter which, if low, can lead to depression and anxiety). So many aspects of your well-being depend upon healthy gut function!

All right, let's jump in.

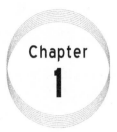

Chapter

1

Toxic Buildup from Food = An Inflamed Gut

Lots of things can lead to gut inflammation. In this chapter, I'll be discussing toxic exposures from genetically modified food, food allergies, and food additives, which can lead to (or perpetuate) gut inflammation.

It can be easy to read this chapter and feel overwhelmed—we cover a lot of information. Again, not all of it may be important for you. We'll recap this at the end of the chapter again, but as you read, please keep in mind that healthy eating is not all that complicated. Most of what I write in this chapter can be encompassed with a few simple rules:

1. **Read the ingredient list.** The shorter the ingredient list, the better. If there is no ingredient list because the product is a whole unprocessed food, that is best of all!
2. **If you don't recognize the ingredient, don't eat it** if you can help it.

3. **Choose foods that will spoil, and eat them before they do.** The less processed, the better. You can usually accomplish this by shopping the perimeter of the grocery store: that's where all the real foods are. The processed junk is usually in the center aisles, in bags, boxes, or cans.

4. **Avoid sugary, processed beverages.** Especially avoid sugary, processed beverages laden with carcinogenic chemicals and food dyes.

If you do just these things, you will likely feel much better. These rules may or may not be enough to get you back to where you want to be, though. For many of you, it will also be necessary to identify and remove food allergens. Before we get into food allergies, let's talk about what allergies are in general.

Allergies

Your immune system is designed to protect your body against harmful substances, such as bacteria, viruses, and foreign substances (allergens). In that sense, allergic responses are not inherently bad. But in a person with allergies, the immune response is exaggerated, and you react to substances that are not generally harmful.

The word "allergies" is kind of a catch-all term, since it can refer to allergic conjunctivitis, atopic dermatitis (eczema), contact dermatitis, hay fever (seasonal allergies), or food or drug allergies, which tend to manifest symptoms all over the body.

Common allergens include medications, dust, food (these reactions can be to the protein, starch, additive, or pesticide on the food), insect bites, mold, pet dander, pollen, hot or cold temperatures, sunlight, or other environmental triggers.

There are actually five kinds of antibodies in your body, but for the purposes of allergy testing, we usually only test two: IgE and IgG. IgE are considered "immediate sensitivity" antibodies, which means your body mounts an immune response to that substance immediately. IgG are "delayed sensitivity" antibodies, which means it may take your body up to 72 hours to mount an immune response.

Skin prick tests are the most common method of allergy testing. This measures IgE ("immediate sensitivity" antibodies). Blood tests can measure either IgE, or IgG. Food allergies are best measured with IgG antibody blood tests, because 80-95% food reactions are of the IgG variety. Blood tests for IgE antibodies are more valuable for environmental allergens such as molds, pet dander, pollens, grasses, dust and the like. These IgE tests are usually covered by insurance, but sometimes you have to fight for it. I will occasionally check IgA as well—these immunoglobulins are only present in the gut, and indicate a gut-only sensitivity, rather than a systemic sensitivity, though most gut inflammation heals by just addressing IgG immunoglobulins.

Allergies of any kind almost always involve the gut. This is because 80% of your immune system resides in your gut. Ideally, your gut should produce a lot of IgA (a lot, but not too much), because it's your first line of defense against any foreign substance. The flora and the lining of your gut need to be healthy in order to produce adequate IgA so that the rest of your body never has to deal with those substances. I test total IgA in stool cultures frequently, in order to identify the integrity of the body's defense system.

Food Allergies

Food allergies are the first thing I think of when I see recurrent sinusitis or upper respiratory infections, asthma, ear infections, eczema, GERD (reflux), heartburn, or psoriasis. In addition to those, though, food allergies can also cause chronic gut issues (gas, bloating, IBS), fluid retention, autoimmunity, behavioral changes (lots of ADD/ADHD kids do much better when allergens are removed), and I've even seen cases where food sensitivities are responsible for hypertension and weight gain.

Nobody is really sure why food allergies are so prevalent, but there are a few theories that make sense to me.

Food allergies could stem from a lack of beneficial flora (probiotics) in our diets. Probiotics are important because they feed on the waste left over after we digest our food, and produce lactic acid, which helps protect our guts against pathogens. We used to get plenty of them by eating raw and fermented foods… but these days, our food is so processed and overheated that there are precious few good flora left over. That sets us up for overgrowth by the bad flora.

Medicines that wipe out gut flora are also suspected of causing allergies. These include antibiotics, certainly, but they also include proton pump inhibitors (such as omeprazole), nSAIDs (like ibuprofen), steroids (like prednisone), birth control, and many others. (More on this in Chapter 4.)

It has also been suggested that genetically modified foods may cause food allergies. If true, this could be because the glyphosate toxin produced by these foods kill off our gut flora, or because the novel components themselves are stimulating our immune systems. It has not been scientifically established that genetically modified foods cause food allergies, but the evidence is strong enough that I avoid them and counsel my patients to do the same. (More on this shortly.)

Really, though, anything causing inflammation in the gut is capable of causing food allergies. This can be a bout of gastroenteritis, trauma, untreated malabsorption syndromes, environmental toxicity, and even chronic stress. If there's inflammation in the lining of the small intestines for any reason, it sets you up to develop sensitivities to foods you could otherwise consume with no problem.

If you think you might have food allergies, you have two choices: 1) see a naturopathic doctor or Functional Medicine doctor who will run an IgG food allergy test for you. 2) Follow an elimination diet. (For more information on how to do this, see Appendix A.)

Leaky Gut Syndrome

Leaky gut syndrome, or Intestinal Hyperpermeability, can be measured with a biomarker called *zonulin*, which is necessary for a tight intestinal barrier. Higher levels in the stool correlate with increased gut permeability, as do the presence of antibodies against it in the blood.[1]

The cells that line your small intestine ought to be tight enough that nothing can get between them without the aid of digestive enzymes. In a leaky gut (or increased intestinal permeability), the junctions between the cells are loose enough that food particles can come in contact with the bloodstream before they've been properly digested. Your blood expects digested nutrients and assumes therefore that the food particles are foreign invaders, and it creates antibodies against them.

Leaky gut also can be the gateway to autoimmune conditions, since allergies and autoimmunity are so closely linked. Allergies are when your immune system thinks a friend is an enemy; autoimmunity is when your immune system thinks *you* are the enemy. The one can set you up for the other.

Zonulin and another protein called *occludin* are the major building blocks of the intestinal tight junctions. Higher levels in the stool, or antibodies in the blood, have been correlated with autoimmune inflammatory bowel conditions such as Crohn's and Ulcerative Colitis, reinforcing the idea that Irritable Bowel Disease is characterized in part by intestinal permeability.[2] Of course, the same association exists with Celiac Disease.[3]

Interestingly, though, increased zonulin levels have also been correlated with other autoimmune conditions that don't necessarily have such a clear "gut" symptom picture, such as Type 1 Diabetes, Ankylosing Spondylitis, Lupus, and Rheumatoid Arthritis.[3]

If you're not sure if you have increased intestinal permeability and don't want to test for food allergies directly, zonulin testing would be the appropriate choice.

Otherwise, you next will need to identify the triggers. That means getting tested for which foods, for you, perpetuate the inflammation in your gut. People who have leaky gut have antibodies (IgG, usually) against the foods they eat the most. Those foods with lower antibody titers can usually be added back into the diet once the gut lining has healed.

For some people, pathogenic bacteria may be an additional culprit (see Chapter 4). This will require a comprehensive stool culture to identify the specific organism and how to get rid of it.

After eradicating pathogenic bacteria, it is necessary to repopulate your gut with good bacteria, since they are a huge part of your immune system.[4] For the most part this is straightforward (unless you also have SIBO, or Small Intestine Bacterial Overgrowth, in which case you'll need to make sure you stick with just the lactobacillus family until it's gone. More on this in Chapter 4).

Before I leave the topic of food allergies and go on to toxins that can contribute to them in general, there are two exceptionally common food allergies that deserve their own mention: dairy and gluten.

Dairy Sensitivity

Our ancestors have been drinking dairy for generations with no problems—but now, all of a sudden, dairy sensitivity is second only to gluten sensitivity. What happened?

For those with an already sensitive gut, dairy is a very common culprit. There are a few possible reasons why.

Dairy is hard to digest. "Sticky" proteins, like gluten, dairy, and eggs (those commonly used in baking) are more likely to cause issues for those without a robust gut to begin with.

Dairy is often full of antibiotics and added hormones. rBGH and rBST are growth hormones given to about one in six dairy cows in the U.S. to increase milk production. These hormones have been known to cause inflammation in the cows' breast tissue, augmenting the need for antibiotics. Dairy cows consume about 70% of this nation's antibiotics both for this reason, as well as to offset the unhealthy conditions in which they are maintained. The reason this is bad news: bacteria are smart. Antibiotics may kill off most of a given strain, but the ones that survive are the ones that are resistant, and then they reproduce... which is the reason why we're having more and more trouble with antibiotic-resistant bacteria these days. Additionally, the milk produced by cows treated with these hormones has a higher concentration of insulin-like growth factor 1 (IGF-1), linked to various kinds of hormonal cancers. rBGH and rBST are banned in Australia, New Zealand, Israel, the EU and Canada... but not in the US.

Dairy products often have a number of additives. Reduced fat or fat free milk has been processed to strip away the cream, which also removes the fat-soluble vitamins A and D. These vitamins must then be added back (which is why you should be leery of any product that says it is "enriched". This term means that vitamins and minerals that were lost during processing were added back. But if a food needs to be enriched in the first place, it's been processed.) Some brands of milk also contain gums like carrageenan, which may cause gut irritation. In general, any product that has been chemically processed is more likely to trigger allergic responses than the original, untampered product.

The two allergens in milk likely to provoke a reaction are the sugar (lactose) and the protein (usually casein, and very rarely whey). The former is found primarily in softer milk products, such as milk and ice cream, while the latter is found primarily in harder milk products, such as hard cheeses, yogurt, and kefir. (If the sensitivity is to the whey component of dairy, then anything that has the liquid part of the milk included will cause problems.)

If you suspect you are sensitive to lactose, casein, or whey, eliminate it for two weeks, and then eat a lot of it for three days. If you're sensitive to it, you'll know pretty quickly after you add it back. However, this will only work if dairy is your only sensitivity. If there are more, the picture will be muddier, at which point you would have to do either a full elimination diet (see Appendix A), or an IgG food sensitivity blood test.

Gluten Sensitivity

The only thing more prevalent than a sensitivity to dairy is a gluten sensitivity. Yet people have been eating wheat since the agricultural age began. So why the sudden explosion in Celiac Disease and gluten sensitivity?

Celiac Disease is an autoimmune condition: it means that in response to the presence of gluten, the body produces antibodies that attack the lining of the small intestine, blunting the villi (tiny finger-like projections where the enzymes live) and preventing absorption of nutrients. An autoimmune condition is when your body attacks itself.

If you have Celiac disease, then yes, I'm afraid you'll have to avoid gluten forever.

Gluten sensitivity, on the other hand, is an allergy—it just means the body produces antibodies (IgG or IgE) against the gluten protein, causing inflammation and poor digestion in the gut. An allergy is when your body attacks something that is ordinarily harmless. In this case, the ordinarily harmless substance is gluten protein which is the glue, or the core binding element, of certain grains (including wheat of course, plus barley, bulgar, couscous, durum, rye, semolina, spelt, and triticale—to name a few).

Statistically, few people had any issues digesting gluten until about fifty years ago, around the end of WWII. Since then, the rate of Celiac Disease has risen over 400%—and that's to say nothing of the many others who are merely gluten sensitive. There seem to be two possible explanations for this: how we grow and process wheat changed around 1960, and how we get the dough to rise (ferment) changed most significantly during the aforementioned war.

Bread rises due to fermentation. Fermentation converts sugar into (in this case) lactic acid and carbon dioxide. The latter is a gas, and that's what makes bread rise.

Up until about a hundred years ago, sourdough was the only kind of bread available, and it is produced in the following manner: flour + water + a sealed container + time –> sourdough starter (consisting of a whole bunch of different strains of bacteria + CO_2 + lactic acid). While the CO_2 makes the bread rise, the lactic acid gives it its characteristic sour flavor. But lactic acid also has three other very important functions: it serves as a natural preservative; it helps to break down certain naturally occurring chemicals (called phytobiotics) that prevent the body from absorbing the nutrients found in the grain; and, most relevant to the topic at hand, lactic acid helps to break down the gluten protein. (Remember, gluten is sticky like glue, and therefore harder to digest on its own, without this assistance.)

Around 1879, however, mass-produced commercial yeast was invented, consisting only of a single strain of yeast (saccharomyces cerevisiae), compared to the veritable zoo of microflora found in sourdough starters. This single yeast ferments the bread much quicker than in sourdough, minimizing or eliminating the benefits of lactic acid. During WWII, this yeast was further refined into granulated active dry yeast, and it was refined further still into instant yeast in the 1970s. (See a correlation in these timelines?)

In 1961, wheat crops also began to be mass-produced. Mass production required the grain to withstand fertilizers, pesticides, heavy machinery, and transcontinental shipping… and in order to achieve such hearty grain, the wheat was bred to contain more gluten than ever before. (Remember, gluten is glue—more gluten means it can take more of a beating.) In order to accommodate the extra gluten in the same amount of "space", though, the trace mineral content in wheat correspondingly declined (and that's before commercial processing strips out the rest of it).

If you *are* gluten sensitive (but do not have Celiac) you can either avoid all gluten-containing food types or replace your usual carbohydrate products with gluten-free products. Unfortunately, most pre-packaged products marketed as "gluten-free" are still highly processed white carbohydrates, which means the carbs turn into sugar as soon as they hit your saliva. You might not have an allergic response to it, but that doesn't make it nutritious.

The good news is that by following traditional grain preparation methods, gluten-containing grains may be tolerable. In 2007, Applied and Environmental Microbiology performed a study demonstrating that while ordinary wheat bread contains gluten levels of 75,000 parts per million, its fermented (sourdough) counterpart instead contained only 12 parts per million—rendering it effectively gluten-free.[20]

Sprouting your grains is another way to achieve essentially the same effect. Raw food naturally contains probiotics and enzymes—enzymes which do essentially the same thing that lactic acid does in terms of breaking down the gluten protein for you. Ezekiel is my favorite brand of sprouted grain products, although you can certainly sprout your own, if you have the time and inclination.

If you have Celiac Disease, you will still need to avoid even sourdough or sprouted grains. But even some of my most gluten-sensitive patients can tolerate sourdough and sprouted grains with no problems.

So much for the two biggest food group issues… on to the discussion of food toxicity in general.

Genetically Modified Organisms (GMOs)

Genetic modification involves taking a gene from one organism, clipping it out of that organism's genome (or *splicing* it) and then inserting it into the genome of a different organism. There's a lot of debate about whether or not that's a good idea. GMOs have been banned to varying degrees in the EU, the UK, Norway, Australia, New Zealand, Thailand, the Philippines, Saudi Arabia, Egypt, Algeria, Brazil, and Paraguay.

The two biggest GMO crops are soybeans (94% of the soybeans in the US are GM) and corn (88% in the US)—if you buy these in the US, they're genetically engineered unless they say otherwise. Other genetically modified crops include cotton, canola (which is made from rapeseed), alfalfa, sugar beets, zucchini, and Hawaiian papaya. These foods are primarily engineered to be herbicide- and insect-resistant, so that they do not need as much pesticide applied to them as non-GM crops, and are resistant to herbicides. Here's the catch, though: there are no long-term human studies to determine safety of these crops, nor are there currently any being done. This is because the FDA considers them to be essentially equivalent to their non-GM counterparts. For that reason, GM foods are not required to be labeled. Most likely, you consume them daily without realizing it, especially if you eat a lot of processed food products.

Despite the official consensus that GM foods are safe for consumption, though, there is cause for caution. The crops often contain a gene from an organism called *Bacillus thuringiensis*, or Bt, which, when expressed, produces a toxin called glyphosate. This is the active ingredient in the insecticide called Round*up*, which kills insects by poking holes in the gut lining. That means these plants actually produce their own Round*up*! According to the EPA, glyphosate is toxic to insects only and has no effect on humans or animals. However, some data links glyphosate with birth defects, miscarriages, infertility, behavioral disorders, and even autism.[5]

Even more compelling to me is the fact that since the 1996 introduction of GM corn and soy into the US, inflammatory gastrointestinal disorders have been on the rise. Admittedly this is only a correlation, and may not be causative. But I can verify from my own practice that leaky gut syndrome is strangely prevalent.

More cause for concern with glyphosate-laden GM foods: glyphosate is a chelator, which means it binds to positively charged elements and compounds (such as trace minerals and nutrients) and doesn't let go. Plants treated with glyphosate may therefore be deficient in nutrients, and the evidence suggests they are primarily low in manganese, zinc, and iron.[21] Although there are studies on both sides of the fence on this issue, it stands to reason that if true, animals eating nutrient deficient plants will then develop nutrient deficiencies themselves. At any rate, it is certainly the case that free-range poultry and grass fed meat are substantially higher in essential fatty acids (EFAs) than their agriculture industry counterparts, and I suspect these issues are related.

So although the official position is that GM foods are safe, we don't know their long-term effects, and there's evidence that they may be harmful. I can attest to the fact that a cleaner diet nearly always dramatically improves my patients' health, although whether this is due to higher quality foods in general or the removal of GM foods specifically, I cannot say.

But in general, my rule is that if the jury's out on safety, avoid it. Be sure to choose organic soy and corn products, OR those that specifically say "non-GMO Project Verified" on the package. Avoid canola oil and cottonseed oil altogether.

Toxins in Meat

If you want to avoid GM foods completely, you will also need to purchase organic meats, because animals bred for slaughter are usually fed the cheaper, chemically laden GM grains. Animal flesh alone can also contain chemicals, metals, and pharmaceuticals.

One of the chemicals found in our meat supply is **ractopamine**. Ractopamine gets added to animal feed in the last few days before slaughter to promote leanness and increase muscle mass. But because the animals consume it so close to the end, as much as 20% of the drug makes its way into the meat we buy at the grocery store. In us, ractopamine has been linked to hyperactivity, behavioral changes, and cardiovascular problems. It has been banned in the EU, Russia, mainland China & the Republic of China (Taiwan).

Non-organic chickens are fed **arsenic** to prevent parasites, bulk up and improve the color of the poultry meat, and decrease the chickens' feed consumption. The result is high levels of inorganic arsenic in the poultry we buy, which is carcinogenic (according to Johns Hopkins).[22] (Seriously, who thought of this?!) Arsenic, sensibly, has been banned from food products in the EU.

Farmed fish, in addition to possibly being fed artificial colors to make their flesh more appetizing, is notoriously high in **heavy metals,** particularly mercury. Fish from the Atlantic are also high in the toxic pesticide PCBs.

Moral of the story: buy your terrestrial meat organic, and your fish wild-caught (and non-Atlantic).

Food Additives

Additives in food contribute to your body's overall toxic load. Even those that do not seem to directly impact the gut can do so, and can contribute to food allergies and leaky gut syndrome. Again, this is because allergies are cumulative: food allergens, environmental allergens, and toxins all can trigger an immune response, resulting in collateral damage. Damage from food additives usually shows up in the gut first, since that is the initial site of insult. I'll list other possible harms caused by each of the additives below, as well; keep in mind that everything is interconnected.

Artificial Food Colors

Artificial food colors are nearly everywhere, and with the petroleum-based FD&C (approved for food, drug, and cosmetic use) colors, often easy to see. These are the colors you associate with candy, brightly colored breakfast cereals, fruit-flavored sodas, rainbow colored frozen treats, and baked goods. FD&C colors are also found in places that you wouldn't necessarily think to look, like fruit snacks and fruit paste products (think bars, tarts, and pies), gelatin desserts, cheeses in all of their forms, sausages, salad dressings, spice mixes, flavored yogurts, frozen meals, and even lemonades. You will be able to recognize these food dyes easily by their names: Blue No. 1 and Blue No. 2, Green No. 3, Red No. 3, Red No. 40, Yellow No. 5, and Yellow No. 6. Collectively these are associated with allergies, brain tumors, bladder and testicular cancer, thyroid tumors, adrenal tumors, kidney tumors, and ADD/ADHD as well as hypersensitivity reactions.[6] For these reasons and more, food dyes are banned in Norway and Austria and contain warnings in the UK and the EU. Those countries use natural food dyes such as beet juice, beta-carotene, blueberry juice concentrate, carrot juice, grape skin extract, paprika, purple sweet potato or corn, red cabbage, and turmeric.

You can safely assume that anything derived from petroleum (i.e. crude oil, also found in gasoline, asphalt, and tar) shouldn't go in your mouth. But just in case you need convincing to stop buying your child's favorite products, let's look at each synthetic color individually:

- **Blue #1** has been shown to trigger allergies.
- **Blue #2** is associated with brain cancer.
- **Green #3** has been associated with thyroid cancer.
- **Red #3** has been recognized by the FDA (Food and Drug Administration) as a carcinogen (cancer-causing substance) for years.
- **Red #40** is commonly contaminated with known carcinogens and is known to cause allergic reactions.
- **Yellow #5** (tartrazine) is especially linked with childhood behavior problems and causes the type of hyperactivity typically associated with ADD/ADHD. On top of that, Yellow #5 is also a known allergen and is routinely contaminated with carcinogens.
- **Yellow #6** is yet another allergenic carcinogen and has been associated with kidney cancer.

Unfortunately, our list of artificial colors doesn't end there. There is another color you need to be aware of; it is found just as often in "natural" products as in the mainstream brands and the amounts and types of products it is put into is staggering. This ubiquitous carcinogen is caramel coloring.[7] Caramel coloring is found in colas, soy and Worcestershire sauces, chocolate-flavored products, beer, and pre-cooked meats, to name just a few items. Again, it is often referred to as natural because it is a sugar-based product, but do not be fooled. Caramel coloring is produced by heating sugar with ammonia or ammonium compounds (you don't cook with ammonia at home, do you?) and is proven to be harmful.

Finally, there is one last color you need to avoid, but you will never see it on a label. Canthaxanthin, which is banned in Australia and New Zealand, is fed to farm-raised salmon in order to restore the pink color they have naturally in the wild. This chemical, although eaten by the fish, is passed directly to you. Canthaxanthin, produced by the pharmaceutical giant Hoffman-La Roche, has been linked to retinal damage.[7] You can easily avoid this toxic color by avoiding farm-raised salmon.

We have seen that artificial colors can directly impact our health, but there is another reason they should be avoided: they convince people to eat processed junk instead of real food. Food dyes add nothing to the flavor of foods, nor do they add nutritional value, but any food product containing artificial coloring almost certainly contains a host of other chemicals as well. Chances are it has also been stripped of any real nutritional value. Do we really want to entice people to eat more junk?

Preservatives

Preservatives are commonly included in processed foods to increase shelf life. They have been associated with allergic reactions, and are stored in body fat (which means it's hard to get rid of them). While you are reading labels, make sure to avoid:

- **BHA** (Butylated hydroxyanisole) and **BHT** (Butylated hydroxytoluene): These are found in prepared and packaged foods, where they are used as a preservative for fat. They have been linked with cancer in rats, mice, and hamsters (so, for good reason, it's a suspected carcinogen in humans). Often these two are used with Propyl Gallate, a preservative of fats as well, also a suspected carcinogen. BHA may also induce allergic reactions and hyperactivity in some sensitive patients. BHA and BHT are banned Japan, in the UK (in infant foods), and in parts of the EU.
- **Sodium Benzoate/Benzoic Acid**: used as a preservative in juices, sodas, and pickles and found in shrimp and fish. When used in beverages containing ascorbic acid (Vitamin C), the two react to form small amounts of benzene, a known carcinogen (cancer-causing agent).
- **Sulfites** (sulfur dioxide, sodium bisulfite): preservatives and bleaching agents in some wine, dried fruit, and processed shrimp and potatoes. These are also sprayed on fruit, veggies, and shrimp, and are associated with asthma. Sulfites can cause severe asthma reactions in sensitive individuals and are also a relatively common trigger for migraines. (You can find all of the aforementioned foods without sulfites, so remember to read your labels.)
- **Trans Fats, aka Partially Hydrogenated Oils**: Trans fat means that hydrogen has been added to a liquid fatty acid to render it solid at

room temperature, increasing its shelf life while also improving texture or "mouth feel." They are found in margarine, shortening, fried foods, and all kinds of processed foods. Once consumed, trans fats are incorporated into your cell walls, causing poor cell membrane and receptor function, and they also increase "bad" cholesterol (LDL) and lower "good" cholesterol (HDL). This contributes to a number of chronic diseases, including heart disease and cancer.[9] Trans fats also lower immune system function and increase insulin resistance. Avoid them completely if at all possible.

- **Sodium nitrate/ sodium nitrite**: The World Cancer Research Fund (WCRF) reviewed more than 7000 clinical studies investigating the links between cancer and diet choices, and concluded the following: "World Cancer Research Fund International recommends avoiding processed meat. This is the conclusion of an independent panel of leading scientists who, following the biggest review of international research ever undertaken, judged the evidence that processed meat increases the risk of bowel cancer to be convincing. This review was done in 2007 and was subsequently confirmed in 2011."[10] Even more compelling to me because my family history includes pancreatic cancer, this study out of the University of Hawaii in 2005 showed that consumption of processed meat products including nitrates and nitrites increased the risk of pancreatic cancer by 68%.[11] Added to preserve color and prolong shelf life, in the body these form carcinogenic (cancer-causing) nitrosamines. Nitrates and/or nitrites can be found in bacon, sausage, hot dogs, beef jerky, lunch meats, and virtually any prepackaged meal containing meat (including pepperoni and salami). The American Cancer Society further notes that high consumption of processed meat over a decade is associated with a 50% increase in the risk for bowel and rectal cancers— where "high consumption" for men is about two slices of bacon OR half a hot dog, 5-6 days per week, and for women, a similar amount 2-3 days per week.[12] This doesn't mean you can't ever have bacon again, but you should be vigilant about the meat products you buy. Health food stores carry bacon (and sausage, and hot dogs) that do not contain nitrates or nitrates, and they'll usually advertise that they are nitrate-free on the front of the package. If not, flip it over and read the ingredients. If it lists nitrates or nitrites, put it back. You can also make your own sausage: free range ground turkey plus a little salt, pepper, sage, and cumin tastes quite similar to the prepackaged varieties. I'd recommend caution with deli meats and processed meat products purchased in restaurants, though—you can easily end up falling into the "high consumption" category if you eat out a lot. When you can opt for unprocessed meats, do so. But if (for instance) your office caters in grinders from the deli for a lunch meeting and your choice is between eating it or going hungry, you can offset the negative impact of the nitrates and nitrites with some extra vitamin C. Ascorbic acid helps block the conversion of nitrates and nitrites to carcinogenic nitrosamines, so it can help protect you in a pinch. So choose a side dish that's rich in Vitamin C (such as broccoli, bell peppers, and citrus fruits), or keep some extra Vitamin C tablets in your purse or your desk, just in case.

Sugar Substitutes

As a general rule, even though excessive sugar is a bad idea (more on this in Chapter 4, the chapter on dysbiosis), if you must sweeten your food it's actually a better idea to use real sugar than the stuff created in a lab. That's because sugar alcohols and artificial sweeteners are your main alternatives. Sugar alcohols such as isomalt, lactitol, sorbitol, mannitol, and xylitol are not as sweet as sugar and often sound like a good sugar alternative because they have a much lower glycemic index and don't cause tooth decay–but the reason they have a lower glycemic index is because they are poorly absorbed. This means that they hang out longer in the gut, increasing the risk of gas and bloating, and in some cases loose stools and diarrhea. It's probably therefore a good idea to not overdo them (particularly if you're reading this book!). Artificial sweeteners you will find on labels are Acesulfame-potassium, Splenda/sucralose, Equal or NutraSweet/aspartame, Sweet 'N Low/saccharin. Collectively these are associated with leukemia, brain tumors, breast cancer, bladder cancer, uterine and ovarian cancer, skin cancer, immune dysfunction, DNA damage, preterm delivery, and neurological problems. Just in case you are thinking to yourself that your favorite sugar-free beverage won't harm you, here are some specifics:

- **Saccharin**: an artificial sweetener found in Sweet and Low, 300-500 times sweeter than sugar. It's associated with bladder cancer when fed to rats in large quantities.
- **Aspartame**: found in Nutrasweet and Equal. It gets metabolized to excitatory amino acids which can lead to neuronal cell death, and has been linked with various neurological diseases such as MS, ALS, and Alzheimer's Disease.[13] It has also been linked to a number of adverse food reactions including headaches, migraines, depression, seizures, weight gain, irritability, insomnia, joint pain, and memory loss.
- **Sucralose**: found in Splenda, which is 600 times sweeter than sugar. Its byproducts are in the same chemical category as certain pesticides (PCBs and DDT), and inconclusive studies suggest that it may cause genetic mutations. High doses have been linked with lower immune function.

Unfortunately, artificial sweeteners aren't even good for your waistline.

At first, this makes no sense—glucose (sugar) can get directly converted into triglycerides which get stored as fat, but artificial sweeteners cannot. The connection between your weight and artificial sweeteners has to do with your microbiome—the good probiotics in your gut.

Your Gut Flora and Your Weight

The Personalized Nutrition Project is a study which (among other things) correlated artificial sweetener consumption with individual gut flora populations.[14] The study found that after even a week of artificial sweetener consumption, the bacterial configurations in the participants' guts had changed, and they started to demonstrate signs of insulin resistance.

In fact, a study from the Journal of the American Geriatrics Society found that over a period of nine years, diet soda intake corresponded to three times the abdominal fat compared to non-diet soda drinkers.[15]

Artificial Sweeteners and Leptin

While sugar has calories and therefore triggers the release of the 'satiety' hormone leptin (which tells your body you're full and to stop eating), artificial sweeteners will stimulate the receptors in your tongue and your brain that say you're eating something sweet, without the caloric payload. This trains you to crave sweeter foods, because artificial sweeteners are between 300-600 times sweeter than sugar. It also lowers the body's satiety response to sweetness. When sugar-like substances don't sustain us, our bodies adapt, lowering the release of leptin and encouraging you to eat more.

The bottom line is that you're not doing your weight a favor with the diet sodas. If that isn't enough, they're laden with phosphoric acid, which acidifies your body and strips minerals from your bones.

If you're looking to wean off a bad habit, you might try health food alternative sodas such as Zevia (which still has artificial colors and chemicals in it, but isn't as bad), or better yet, switch to diluted fruit juice (you can dilute it with carbonated water if you're craving the fizz). Or just go straight to flavored carbonated water, or to unsweetened iced tea.

Individual Additives

You now know the major groups (artificial colors, preservatives, sugar substitutes) of additives that need to be avoided, but there are a few more that don't fit neatly into a category and must be remembered by name.

- **Monosodium Glutamate/MSG**: This is used as a flavor enhancer in various processed foods. It is especially common in Chinese food prepared in restaurants, where it is added to increase the salty flavor of protein. MSG is primarily a problem only for individuals who are sensitive (sensitivities include headaches and migraines, nausea, burning sensations, increased heart rate, weakness, and wheezing or difficulty breathing) or allergic (chest tightness, diarrhea, headaches, and flushing).

However, large amounts have been associated with neural damage in animal studies.[16]

- **Olestra/Olean**: These fat substitutes are found in "fat-free" chips primarily. (Note: any packaged food that boasts "fat-free," "sugar-free" or "fortified" usually makes up for it with a cocktail of chemicals. AVOID.) Like their "sugar-free" cousins, sugar alcohols, olestra manages to taste like fat without the same impact on the body because it's indigestible. Side effects therefore include diarrhea, cramps and leaky bowels, as well as poor absorption of fat soluble vitamins such as A, D, E and K. As if that wasn't bad enough, in 2011, Purdue University demonstrated that rats fed potato chips made with Olean actually gained weight. Olestra and Olean are banned in the UK and Canada.[17]

- **Potassium Bromate**: Potassium bromate gets added to commercial bread products because it improves the volume of bread by helping the dough hold together and rise higher, and it is also approved by the FDA for use in malting barley. Bromate usually breaks down into bromide, which does not appear to be harmful. However, bromate itself is a carcinogen in animals. Some studies indicate that potassium bromate may be carcinogenic, and link it to nervous system and kidney damage.[18] Potassium Bromate is also one of the possible contributors to the hypothyroidism epidemic. Due to the location of bromine on the periodic table, it behaves very much like iodine, thus potentially interfering with the production of thyroid hormone. It is banned in Canada, China and the EU.

- **Brominated Vegetable Oil**: BVO shows up in a number of beverages, such as Mountain Dew, Fresca, and some flavors of Powerade (though it was recently removed from Gatorade). It acts as an "emulsifier," helping to distribute the flavor and prevent layers of chemical separation. Again, bromine is linked to thyroid trouble (see above), tremors, depression, confusion, and several kinds of cancer (according to Mayo Clinic). Brominated Vegetable Oil is banned in the EU and Japan.

- **Phosphoric Acid**: an additive in sodas that strips your body, and your bones, of essential nutrients. Phosphoric acid is added to soda to give it a "tangy" flavor, and it makes it very acidic. Your blood, however, has to maintain a very specific pH... and if you ingest something very acidic, it has to "buffer" that acidity with minerals, which it strips from your bones. This can set you up for osteoporosis.

Non-Toxic Additives You May Want to Watch Out For

Some food additives truly are natural and don't really carry a toxic burden. For health reasons, though, you should know about them so you use them responsibly or identify a possible sensitivity. These are two of the most common:

- **Caffeine**: Although a little caffeine isn't necessarily bad, too much definitely is. Caffeine doesn't directly increase adrenaline, but it does allow it to work unhindered. This can mean increased blood pressure, heart rate, palpitations, blood flow to the muscles, irritability and/or anxiety, as well as decreased blood flow to the brain.[19] This, again, can contribute to impaired concentration and focus if you overdo it. Too much caffeine can also contribute to adrenal fatigue, and weakened adrenals can lead to a whole host of problems, including increased susceptibility to food allergies and leaky gut syndrome. Depending on how exhausted you are, consuming caffeine to keep going is like whipping a dead horse.
- **Salicylates**: these are chemically similar to aspirin, and so people with allergies to aspirin may not tolerate them well. They are found in cake mixes, sodas, dried fruits and berries, gum, pudding, and ice cream, and they are also used to enhance the flavor of certain spices.

We've covered a lot and at this point you may be wondering if there is anything you *can* eat. There is. To simplify, you can sum up almost everything we have covered as follows: if it contains a chemical you don't recognize, do not put it in your mouth. Your awareness of the toxic chemicals in our food supply is important! If the FDA does not ban these chemicals, it's up to us to vote with our dollars. If we stop buying foods full of chemicals, companies will eventually stop producing them. Many of the larger grocery chains such as Wal-Mart and Costco have begun to carry organic, nitrate- and nitrite-free, free range, and other healthy food products. Our good health often depends on knowing whether a product is beneficial or toxic.

Understanding Product Claims

How do you really know what goes into a box of cereal or other food package? What do all of those impressive-sounding labels really mean?

When you start shopping for non-toxic food products, you will quickly notice that there is a very large supply of foodstuffs that claim to be health-promoting in some way. Often they are packaged in green or brown and cost considerably more that their shelf-mates. What do all of these claims mean, though? Are they really good for us? The short answer is "maybe." You will still need to do some label detective work. If it says "fat-free," "sugar-free," or anything else "-free," be skeptical. And probably don't eat it.

- **Natural or Organic**: Natural just means the product does not include synthetic or artificial ingredients. That's good in the sense that you want to avoid consuming as many chemicals as possible, because, as you know, many of them have been linked with a number of illnesses. Organic means the food is grown without fertilizers, insecticides, herbicides, or growth hormones according to USDA standards. Sometimes it's worth it to pay more for organic and sometimes it isn't, based on the pesticide load of the inorganic version of the food. In general, for fresh produce, you want to buy any of the "dirty dozen" fruits and veggies organic, while you can buy nonorganic on the "clean fifteen" if budget is a concern. You can find the current list of both here: http://www. ewg.org/foodnews/summary/. It gets a little trickier to work out with packaged goods, but at least organic processed foods containing corn or soy derivatives (which most of them do) will not be genetically modified.
- **Lean and Extra Lean**: These terms apply to meat, poultry, and fish. Lean means there's less than 10 grams of fat, 4.5 grams or less of

saturated fat, and 95 mg cholesterol per 100 grams. Extra lean means less than 5 gm fat, less than 2 grams saturated fat, and less than 95 mg cholesterol per 100 grams. It's a good idea to choose lean meats, as they decrease the risk of cancer otherwise associated with other meats. But it's most important to choose organic and free range meats if at all possible, because free range meats contain a better ratio of omega-3 to omega-6 (decreasing the risk of many inflammatory diseases), and organic meats do not contain growth hormones.

- **Enriched and Fortified**: Both of these terms mean that vitamins and minerals were added to the food, but fortified means more of the nutrients naturally found in the food were added, while enriched means that vitamins and minerals that were lost during processing were added back. But don't think that the food itself is healthy just because the company added a few extra nutrients. If a food needs to be enriched in the first place, it's processed, and processing leads to a number of other problems. Also beware of the high sugar content commonly found in processed foods.

- **Heart Healthy**: This is a bit of a catch-all term, meaning the food is low in calories, whole grain, fat free, and/or made with oil instead of saturated fat. The label is usually unregulated though, so you should take it with a grain of salt (no pun intended).

- **Low Fat and Fat Free**: Low fat means three grams of fat or less per serving size. Fat free means what it sounds like: only traces of fat exist in the food or none at all. If you choose these foods because you're trying to lose weight, beware that fat free does NOT mean low calorie. In fact, for purposes of weight loss it's more important to avoid sugar and processed carbohydrates than fat.

- **Whole Grain**: This means that all three major components of the grain kernel remain in the food: bran, germ, and endosperm. The bran contains fiber and B vitamins, magnesium, phosphorus, iron and zinc. The germ contains Vitamin E, selenium, thiamine, iron, magnesium, phosphorus, zinc, and protein. The endosperm contains protein and carbohydrates. When grains are milled, they lose the bran and the germ, retaining only the protein and carbs from the endosperm. The lack of fiber in processed grains means that the remaining carbs hit your bloodstream almost immediately, and they act basically just like sugar. Additionally, the loss of the bran and germ removes most of the nutritional value of the grain. So whole grains are most definitely a better idea than processed. But be aware: if they do not say 100% whole grain, most likely the product is a mixture of whole grains and refined grains, which means the glycemic index will still be quite high. You can tell whether this is the case by reading the ingredient list: if it says "enriched" next to the flour, it's refined.

- **Gluten Free**: Gluten is a protein found in the germ (see above) of wheat, rye, barley, and several other grains. As mentioned earlier, gluten intolerance and Celiac Disease are both relatively common, and especially for Celiac patients, total gluten avoidance is critical. That said, if you are not gluten sensitive, you don't really need to avoid it and eating gluten free some of the time will have no benefit. However, most non-organic wheat has been sprayed heavily with Round-*Up* prior to harvest. It is therefore a good idea to buy any gluten-containing products organic, though, to avoid the glyphosate contamination.

Sodium: To Avoid or Not To Avoid?

In addition to the previously listed product label claims, you will undoubtedly see a number of products advertising that they are low in sodium. Is that better for you? It's a common belief that too much sodium is bad for your health, and especially your blood pressure. Let's take a look at where this idea comes from.

Any living system seeks to create balance, or homeostasis. One aspect of this is electrolyte balance. Sodium is the most abundant electrolyte in the body, followed by chloride (not surprising, since in table salt they come together). Your body balances electrolyte concentrations found in different compartments by shifting around water content, because water can pass through membranes (while electrolytes can't, not without assistance). Therefore, when sodium concentration on one side of a membrane is higher than on the other, water content follows in order to balance it out. If you've just recently eaten a lot of sodium, the concentration will be higher in your bloodstream, so the water will flow out of your cell membranes and into your bloodstream to balance it out. More water = higher blood volume = higher blood pressure.

But the flip side is true too. If you've been under a lot of stress for a long period of time, you might notice that the room goes dark for a few seconds when you stand up too quickly. This is called orthostatic hypotension, and it occurs because your adrenal glands produce several hormones. One of them is cortisol, responsible for most of the classic symptoms of adrenal fatigue. But another is called aldosterone. Aldosterone reabsorbs sodium and exchanges it for potassium at the level of the kidneys. Again, water follows sodium. So if your adrenals are too tired to make enough aldosterone, you'll likely notice that your blood pressure will go down. This means your heart will have to work extra hard to get the lower blood volume all the way up to your head when you stand up too fast. People in this position will sometimes find that they crave salt… and for good reason. The body is trying to get that blood volume back up.

Sodium-containing foods are very acidifying to the body. This doesn't mean that they make your blood acidic—if that happened, you'd be dead. What it does mean is these foods overtax the buffering system your body employs to maintain the pH of your blood within a very narrow range. But there's no such thing as a "free lunch"… an overtaxed buffering system means overworked kidneys, potential kidney stones, and sometimes osteoporosis. It may even predispose you to cancer. Anybody who's ever tried to drink seawater knows that salt makes you thirsty, for the same balancing reasons mentioned above. But you can fall off the "other side of the horse," as it were, by drinking only distilled or Reverse Osmosis (RO) water. Electrolytes in the proper balance help the cells actually get and stay hydrated, rather than flushing right through you.

Processed and prepackaged foods are, for the most part, high in sodium. (Side note here: MSG, or monosodium glutamate, binds to sodium receptors in your taste buds and "tricks" your brain into thinking the food is saltier than it really is. Even if you are not actually allergic or sensitive to MSG, training your taste buds to crave too much salt perpetuates this problem.) Yes, you need sodium to maintain adequate blood volume and hydration status, but there is most definitely too much of a good thing, and we're there. This is why many people who have hypertension, kidney stones, and osteoporosis will notice that when they start watching their sodium intake, health indices will improve.

But historically, the bulk of our diets didn't consist of prepackaged foods, and our palates didn't come to expect excessively salty flavors. In those days, natural salt, containing a complex variety of other minerals besides just sodium, was extremely valuable for its ability to both preserve and bring out the flavor in savory foods. Unlike the processed table salt we're familiar with today, natural salt such as sea salt is a good source of sodium, in the proper balance with other electrolytes.

The Take-Home Message: Eating for Health

If you are wondering if there is anything left to eat or drink, just take a breath and know that eating healthy really isn't that hard—most of our ancestors had it figured out! All it takes is a little common sense. If you feel overwhelmed at the grocery store, let's revisit the simple rules we discussed at the beginning of the chapter.

1. **Read the ingredient list.** The shorter the ingredient list, the better. The best food is the one with no ingredient list at all, because the product is a whole, unprocessed food.
2. **If you don't recognize the ingredient, don't put it in your body.**
3. **Choose foods that will spoil, and eat them before they do.** The less processed, the better.
4. **Avoid sugary, processed beverages.** Especially avoid artificially sweetened, processed beverages laden with carcinogenic chemicals and food dyes.

Above all, remember that what you choose to feed your family does make a difference!

Chapter 2

Toxic Buildup from Western Society = Gut Inflammation

O ur bodies can be overwhelmed by the assault of chemicals in modern living. Our food, furnishings, housing, cosmetics, cleaning products, paper products, cars, and all other belongings carry the stamp of the chemical industry. I won't argue that these products are bad, because they have allowed us to live in comfort and accomplish great things. But for many of us, our livers are simply not up to the task of filtering these extreme levels of pollutants. If the liver can't keep up, these toxins end up in the bloodstream, leading to a toxic body burden. A backed up liver also nearly always leads to a damaged gut, poor nutrient absorption, and often food allergies and leaky gut syndrome.

Many of these toxic exposures happen within our houses or places of work, or because we choose products and services that are harmful to us. By understanding the dangers of everyday items and seeking appropriate substitutes, you will be able to avoid the things that don't have a risk:benefit ratio that you are comfortable with.

Once again, there is a lot of information in this chapter, and very likely more detail than you will need. So as you read, keep in mind that if you follow this basic rule, you will go a long way toward reducing your overall body burden:

Buy personal care and household cleaning products with a short list of ingredients, all of which you recognize.

Remember, too, that toxins have an additive effect. Your liver is like a big trash bucket. It can accommodate a certain number of toxins just fine, and you will never know the difference. The problem comes in once the bucket is full; then the toxic elements the liver can't get to fast enough will spill over into the bloodstream, recirculate, and trigger immune responses. The "tipping point" where this happens is different for everyone. If you have had a major toxic exposure, you will probably need to follow some of the cleansing techniques at the end of this chapter to "dump the bucket". If you have not, eliminating even a few of the toxins mentioned in this chapter may be enough.

Do what you can do, try not to get overwhelmed, and when in doubt. remember the rule: short ingredient list, nothing you don't recognize.

Endocrine Disrupting Chemicals

By far the most common illness-inducing pollutants are endocrine disrupting chemicals. They are *everywhere,* and the manufacturers of those chemicals churn out millions of gallons every day.

Endocrine disrupting chemicals can screw up your hormones. Many of them are estrogenic, and the vast majority of female endocrine issues I've seen stem from estrogen dominance relative to progesterone. Quite a few of these also disrupt the thyroid, which makes sense—hypothyroidism has swelled to near-epidemic proportions as well. It is important to learn where these chemicals are hiding, because they are never advertised. (Hypothyroidism can cause constipation, leading to bloating, slow bowel transit and even SIBO. Female hormone imbalance often leads to gut symptoms as well. More on this in Chapter 6.)

You have probably heard of the chemical **Bisphenol A (BPA)** and know that the FDA has banned inclusion of BPA in baby bottles. But you may not be aware that the current FDA position states that BPA is safe.[8] BPA is used in hard plastics and in the resin lining the insides of most food and beverage cans, and the FDA continues to hold that the BPA lining food and beverage cans is not a health concern. However, it has been demonstrated that BPA binds to and stimulates the estradiol receptor, tricking the body into thinking estrogen levels are higher than they are.[9] Unfortunately, some plastics labeled BPA-free have similar effects, as well.[10] Avoid BPA by choosing fresh over canned foods and avoiding the use of hard plastics.

Like BPA, **phthalates** have been in the news repeatedly, and you have most likely heard of them. Primarily found in plastics to increase flexibility, phthalates are not only estrogenic, they have been found to increase apoptosis, or programmed cell death, particularly in testicular cells. (Apoptosis is the normal mechanism for a mutated cell to self-destruct. When upregulated, this means healthy cells undergo destruction unnecessarily.) The phthalates are not bonded to the plastics and are fat-soluble, and they therefore leech easily into fatty foods packaged in flexible plastic wrapping. Cosmetics and personal care products also deliver a dose of phthalates topically. Overall, phthalates are linked to breast cancer, birth defects, low sperm count, obesity, diabetes, and thyroid problems. To avoid phthalates, store your food and beverages in glass rather than plastic as much as possible, read labels for personal care items to make sure phthalates are not on the list, make sure you use glass or stainless steel water bottles, and NEVER microwave food with plastic wrap on top! (If you must microwave, use paper towels to avoid splatter instead.)

Polybrominated diphenyl ethers (PBDEs), unfortunately, are just as pervasive as BPA and phthalates. PBDEs are found throughout homes because they are used in fire retardants that are applied to foam furniture, carpets, and a variety of other products. PBDEs also don't break down very well and therefore bioaccumulate. They're everywhere, and they have been shown to decrease fertility and disrupt thyroid activity. Hopefully laws will better protect us in the future and render these less ubiquitous. These can be avoided with very expensive specialty furniture or alternative-type furnishings, but in the meantime, honestly

I just don't worry about it. (You can easily get obsessive about avoiding every possible toxic exposure, and that can be even more damaging than the chemicals, if there's little you can do about it.)

Case Study:

Patricia came to me with a bizarre rash, bloating, constipation, and diarrhea, food sensitivities to nearly everything, and crushing fatigue, despite being on more than a full thyroid replacement dose. She was also on more than a full adrenal replacement dose of hydrocortisone. When I asked when everything started, she told me that it was about two years before, when she and her husband had moved into a new house. New homes, or recently renovated homes, are notoriously contaminated with chemicals such as PBDEs, VOCs from paint, etc.

We put her on a protocol to eliminate the solvents, which tend to hide in the fat cells—so the protocol involved a far infrared sauna (to release the solvents into her bloodstream), alternating hot and cold (constitutional hydrotherapy) to flush the solvents into her organs of elimination, castor oil packs to help her liver dump into her colon, and colonics to trigger bile dumping and eliminate the solvents from her body entirely. She was to perform this protocol a minimum of three times per week for a minimum of six weeks.

We also did food allergy testing in office, but I knew it would come back with a sensitivity to almost everything. I also changed the way she dosed her hydrocortisone to three times daily instead of twice daily, and I switched her from Levothyroxine to the natural thyroid, NatureThroid, but at an equivalent dose. Then I gave her a lab requisition form to re-check her thyroid in 6 more weeks. When Patricia returned three weeks later to review the food allergy results, she told me she was already feeling better: the fatigue had begun to lift just a little, and the rash was mostly gone.

Sure enough, her IgG food allergies were off the charts. The scale goes from 0 to 6, so I took out only the ones in the 5-6 range (which was still a list of about nine foods). I also gave her glutamine to heal up the gut lining, as the food for the small intestine, and probiotics to help her repopulate with the good stuff.

Three weeks later, Patricia returned to follow up on her labs. They showed that her thyroid was actually suppressed, so we lowered her NatureThroid dose. She said her fatigue had improved dramatically, so much so that she had cut her hydrocortisone dose in half on her own. The rash had disappeared completely, and her gut had already responded to treatment (which I told her was unusual—most people don't notice much difference until about week 4 on an allergy elimination protocol). The bloating had vanished, and her bowel movements returned to normal.

Three weeks after that, Patricia had stopped her hydrocortisone entirely. She'd gotten busy and stopped doing the detox protocol because she didn't think she needed it anymore. We transitioned her to a rotation diet in which she continued to avoid the highest food allergens except very occasionally, and she rotated some of the lower offenders such that she at least was not consuming them daily. Eventually, she even got off of thyroid medication altogether!

Can you see from Patricia's story how interconnected the body's systems are? All of her symptoms ultimately went back to her body's reaction to solvents. Not everyone is as sensitive as Patricia, of course—her husband and children didn't have nearly the reaction to their new home that she did. The timing of her symptoms clued me in to the fact that her liver had either already been at capacity to begin with, or else it wasn't quite as efficient as those of her family members.

Used as much as PBDEs are **organophosphate pesticides**. Organophosphate pesticides are some of the most common pesticides in use today, and they are neurotoxic to insects. Unfortunately they're neurotoxic to us as well. For that reason, OP use has been banned in most residential areas, but they're still commonly used on fruits and veggies, and are also used in plastics and as solvents. They've been linked with low testosterone and thyroid disruption. Avoid them by buying the Dirty Dozen fruits and veggies organic, limiting your exposure to solvents, and finding alternatives to plastic.

PFCs, or perfluorinated chemicals, are widely-used endocrine disrupting chemicals. Used in non-stick cookware and water-resistant coatings, these pretty much never break down in the environment. They have also been linked to low sperm count, kidney and thyroid disease. Instead of the non-stick variety, choose stainless steel pots and pans—I know they're a pain to clean, but they're much safer. Also try to limit your use of disposable tableware and to-go containers.

PFCs are not the only toxin associated with disposable products. **Dioxins** are a class of chemicals that are mostly byproducts of the production of pesticides, waste incineration, and bleaching paper pulp. Unfortunately, they're also tenacious—once they show up in the environment, they're not readily broken down. They hide in fat cells, and most of our exposure actually comes from animals: that is, the animals accumulate them in their fat and then we eat the animal, or drink its milk. Once they're in our bodies, dioxins have half-lives of years. These, too, have endocrine disrupting properties, and have been linked to low sperm count and various kinds of cancer. Avoid these by minimizing agriculture industry dairy and meat. Instead choose organic whenever possible. Also avoid disposable wood pulp products that have extended contact with your skin (think diapers and feminine care products) that do not specifically say that they are dioxin-free.

Atrazine, like dioxin, is another food-contaminating endocrine disrupter. An herbicide used on most corn crops in the US, Atrazine is now a common contaminant in drinking water. Research shows that exposure to even a small amount can turn male frogs into hermaphrodites (with viable eggs!) It is banned in the EU but commonly used in the US and in Australia. Avoid it by choosing organic fruits and veggies, and drinking filtered water (not from a plastic bottle!)

Perchlorate is yet another drinking water contaminant. Referring to a salt with the polyatomic anion perchloric acid, it does occur both naturally and industrially, as it's used in rocket fuel. Because the mineral occurs naturally, it can contaminate drinking water. It inhibits the thyroid's ability to obtain iodine, a necessary mineral for thyroid hormone production, and was therefore once considered the standard of care for hyperthyroidism. However, given today's epidemic of hypothyroidism, it's wise to avoid it and choose filtered water whenever possible.

Finally, **glycol ethers** are used as solvents in paint, cleaning solutions, brake fluid, and cosmetics (Did you see that? Cosmetics!) These may lower sperm count, decrease fertility, and they have been associate with allergies and asthma. Avoid them by choosing cleaning products that lack 2-butoxyethanol (EGBE) and methoxydiglycol (DEGME), carefully reading cosmetic labels, and choosing no-VOC paint products.

Obesogens: Chemicals That Make Us Fat

Some of the endocrine disrupting chemicals that we have already discussed have earned themselves a special term: *obesogens*. That is because they make us obese. Weight gain often leads to insulin resistance and metabolic syndrome; metabolic syndrome means high blood sugar, among other things, which very often leads to dysbiosis and gut inflammation.

In the last decade or so, animal studies have increasingly indicated that certain chemicals, particularly those already known to be endocrine (hormone) disruptors, can lead to obesity.

Research started with tributylin (TBT), used to paint the underside of ships to prevent barnacles from growing there. The studies showed that TBT activates a fatty acid receptor, which regulates fat cell development. Sure enough, animals who had been exposed to TBT, particularly in utero, grew up to be fatter than their ancestors.[1]

Other endocrine disrupting chemicals that behave this way include the pesticides DDT and PCBs, tolyfluanid, a flame retardant called 2,2',4,4'-tetrabrominated diphenyl ether, or BDE-47, phthalates, found in plastics, and triflumizole, a fungicide.[2] You can avoid PCBs by buying your fish wild-caught, and DDT, triflumizole, and tolyfluanid by buying the Dirty Dozen fruits and veggies organic. The list is updated yearly on the Environmental Working Group website.

Avoid phthalates by choosing glass or pyrex storage containers rather than plastic ware, choose glass or stainless steel water bottles instead of plastic ones, and skip the plastic wrap in the microwave—use a paper towel instead to avoid splatter.

Some obesogens can make you fat by altering levels of cortisol. Cortisol is an adrenal hormone that helps us deal with stress—but it also breaks down glycogen and initiates gluconeogenesis in the liver, both of which increase circulating glucose. Glucose (sugar) in excess of our metabolic needs then gets stored as fat, and this leads to both obesity and insulin resistance. (By the way, chronically elevated cortisol can set you up for leaky gut syndrome, too.)

Obesogens that can make you fat via excess cortisol include DDT, PCBs, and tolyfluanid again, as well as endrin (another pesticide), and Bisphenol A (BPA) and phthalates, both found in plastics.[2, 3] BPA also is found in the lining of canned foods.

You can avoid BPA by skipping canned foods (even those that boast they are BPA-free have a chemical in the bisphenol family instead).

Some obesogens cause insulin resistance more directly, by decreasing the production of members of the insulin signaling cascade. (What that means: signaling in your body is kind of like a Rube Goldberg machine, where one thing triggers another triggers another.) Tolyfluanid, again, is a chemical that does this.[4]

Xenoestrogens, or chemicals that act like estrogen in the body, can also pack on the pounds. BPA can do this—but the heavy metals cadmium, arsenic, and lead, which have their own section in this chapter, can do the same.[5] Unfortunately, xenoestrogens can be found in great abundance in our modern world. Sources include soft plastics (phthalates), canned food (bisphenol A), pesticides (dioxins, atrazine, organophosphates), agriculture industry dairy and meat (dioxins, growth hormones), foam furniture (polybrominated biphenyl ethers), carpeting (polybrominated biphenyl ethers), metal amalgams (mercury), non-stick cookware (perfluorinated chemicals), water-resistant coatings (perfluorinated chemicals), and cleaning products (glycol ethers).

If you are wondering where the United States Environmental Protection Agency (EPA) comes in with all this, it turns out the EPA has not attempted to ban any chemicals at all since the 1980s. This is apparently because despite a decade of lobbying to ban asbestos, a known carcinogen, they were ultimately overruled by bureaucratic red tape.[6]

So it's up to you and me to limit our exposure to these chemicals. More severe exposures, or people whose livers are not as efficient at detoxing as they should be, may need a full cleanse protocol. But for most of us, avoidance goes a long way.

Heavy Metals and Toxic Elements

Only slightly less prevalent than their chemical cousins are the heavy metals. Because heavy metals readily bioaccumulate like the toxins mentioned above, it is imperative that you understand that we truly live in a toxic world. Thankfully, according to naturopathic theory, if you remove the obstacles to cure and give the body what it needs to heal itself, then within reason, it will.

Toxins of all kinds fall under the category of "obstacles to cure," which means we've got to do two things: limit our ongoing exposure, and get rid of the toxins that have already accumulated in our tissues.

Heavy metals are getting more and more attention these days as obstacles to cure and even as causes of certain illnesses. Here's a quick breakdown of the most common offenders.

Lead is found in old paint, solder in plumbing (and therefore in drinking water), and even in some herbal remedies imported from overseas. Lead exposure can also be geographical or occupational (living near or working in a lead smelter or lead mine, welding, construction, and manufacture of certain products such as glass, vinyl mini-blinds, and ceramic glaze). Lead initially gets stored in the bones, and is released when bone turnover increases (such as in pregnancy and menopause). It can disrupt the HPA (Hypothalamus-Pituitary-Adrenal) axis, making it harder to deal with stress. In children, lead has been linked with learning and developmental disabilities including lower IQ and ADD. It is also associated with other neurological problems such as depression and anxiety, Alzheimer's, and Parkinson's Disease. It can cause high blood pressure, often poorly or unresponsive to medication. Again, filter your water. (And don't allow young children to eat the paint, if you live in an old house. Probably don't let them eat the paint anyway, that's a good rule of thumb.) Also, if you purchase herbal remedies imported from overseas, make sure you do so from a trusted brand that tests for heavy metals and certifies their products are uncontaminated.

You are probably also aware that **mercury** is a relatively common metal that can have toxic effects. Unfortunately, you may not be aware that minuscule mercury exposures are not as safe as you have been told, and may be causing you significant problems. Mercury is found in farmed or Atlantic fish, and also in dental amalgams. (If you have a mouth full of mercury fillings, you can let off enough mercury vapor every time you chew that your mouth will exceed OSHA standards for acceptable levels!) Mercury used to be used as a preservative in vaccines called thimerosol, but thimerosol has been eliminated from most vaccines now except for the influenza vaccine. (It is possible to get flu vaccines without thimerosol, though.) Mercury concentrates in the nervous system and is linked to a variety of neurological disorders. It disrupts steroid hormones and potentially interferes with insulin production. It even eats up your body's antioxidant reserves, leaving you vulnerable to oxidative damage. This is probably why mercury has been linked to an increased risk of cardiovascular disease. Mercury also inhibits your body's ability to make ATP (adenosine triphosphate, the energy currency of the body). To avoid mercury, choose wild-caught or Pacific fish, and avoid tuna, orange roughy, swordfish, shark, halibut, and snapper. Consider eating cod, whitefish, tilapia, ocean perch, shrimp, flounder, scallops, clams, and catfish instead. And if you have amalgams and have the money, consider looking into a biological or holistic dentist to replace the fillings.

Aluminum is another metal that we have been told is safe. It is not. Aluminum is found in pans for cooking, "tin" foil, aluminum-based antiperspirants, antacids and many other over-the-counter medications, and in processed foods using baking powder (not baking soda—these are different) and self-rising flour (those that don't include yeast). Examples include processed cheese and cheese products, cake mixes, pancake mixes, rising flours, and frozen dough. Aluminum has also replaced mercury in most vaccines as a preservative. Aluminum concentrates in the lungs, bones, and nervous system and there is evidence that aluminum may be correlated with the rise in autism.[7] Aluminum has also been linked to breast cancer, kidney failure, dementia, Alzheimer's, MS, ALS, and Parkinson's disease. Be sure to choose non-aluminum based antiperspirants—or just choose a deodorant and not an antiperspirant at all, if you can handle it. Certain natural deodorants work quite well when used in conjunction with a healthy, non-toxic lifestyle. (Remember that sweat is one of the body's mechanisms to eliminate toxins—the more toxic you are, the smellier you tend to be!)

Also avoid over-the-counter meds that contain aluminum, including antacids. Aluminum is sometimes listed as an active and sometimes as an inactive ingredient, so read your labels. (You shouldn't need to be taking antacids regularly anyway. If you are, you're just treating the symptom, not the cause—which, for heartburn and reflux, is very often food allergies. See Chapter 1.)

If you are having symptoms, you might consider replacing your aluminum pans. Cast iron or stainless steel are a good choice. They're harder to scrub clean, though. The new ceramic non-stick pans also seem to be a safe alternative to Teflon.

Finally, avoid products containing baking powder in the ingredient list, unless specifically stated that it does not contain aluminum. If they don't say that it is aluminum-free, assume that it isn't. The same goes for self-rising flour. (Generally you shouldn't be eating processed foods anyway, if I haven't said that enough.)

You may not think you need to worry about **arsenic** because you consider it an outright poison, but it is found in more places than just in your (non-organic) chicken. Arsenic is also found in seafood, herbicides, and drinking water. Arsenic is a carcinogen that interferes with the regulation of cortisol and can lead to the symptoms of high cortisol and/or low cortisol. Be sure to buy your chicken organic, and choose wild-caught, Pacific seafood. And again, filter your water.

Found mostly in cigarettes, **cadmium** also concentrates in the water, air, and soil especially in industrial areas where smelting and refining occurs—thus, it can be found in the food supply in those regions. It is also used in the manufacture of batteries or plastics. Cadmium is a carcinogen that concentrates in the kidneys, liver, and pancreas, but is easily absorbed through the lungs and can lead to kidney failure, gout, and loss of sense of smell. It is hard to avoid industrial cadmium pollution, but you can certainly stop smoking and limit your exposure to second-hand smoke to avoid much of it.

Fluoride comes from the element fluorine—the most reactive element on the periodic table. Because of this, too much of it can interrupt some of the body's critical activities and act as a poison. Fluoride concentrates in bones, and because of this, too much fluoride can actually weaken teeth and bones. It has been linked with osteosarcoma, a very aggressive bone cancer. Cosmetically, excessive fluoride can cause enamel fluorosis (mottling or white streaks across the teeth). Fluoride is found in toothpaste and dental care products and is also added to the water supply of many municipalities. You can avoid it by filtering your water and choosing fluoride-free dental products (other toothpastes plus the physical action of brushing will clean your teeth just fine).

To minimize the heavy metal exposures that are out of your control, make sure you're getting your daily dose of antioxidants. These will both counter the effects of some heavy metals, and improve your body's natural detoxification mechanisms. Make sure, too, that you're getting your daily dose of chlorophyll. This means eating lots of greens—the darker the better! It is also important to make sure you're getting your daily dose of fiber. Fiber helps to bind and eliminate toxins of all kinds. Whole grains and veggies are a great source. And, finally, don't forget to drink plenty of water! This flushes out your cells, and helps to prevent constipation, which will clearly impede toxic elimination.

Sulfur Intolerance

A quick interlude here: if you have heavy metal toxicity, you might think you're experiencing lots of allergies, when in reality, your issue might be sulfur intolerance.

From a nutritional standpoint, the primary reason we care about sulfur is because the second phase of liver detoxification (rendering a toxic molecule less harmful) requires sulfur. Three of the liver's Phase II Detoxification processes, sulfation, glucoronidation, and glutathione-S-transferase, all require sulfur. Glutathione is also most powerful antioxidant in the body, comprised of three amino acids: cysteine (which contains sulfur), glutamine, and glycine.

You need sulfur. You can't completely avoid it.

And yet, some people can't tolerate sulfur in large quantities. Sulfur sensitivity can lead to recurrent yeast overgrowth (see Chapter 4), despite diet restrictions and antifungals. Symptoms of excess sulfur also look a lot like a histamine reaction, including hives, itchiness, asthma, headaches, nausea, fatigue, flushing, and brain fog.

For people who have a sensitivity to sulfur (or sulfites, which are sulfur atoms complexed with three oxygen atoms), foods and supplements high in the sulfur-containing amino acids can be a problem. Foods high in thiols seem to be especially troublesome. Here's a list of high thiol foods:

- **Veggies:** artichokes, asparagus, beans, peas, and lentils, all cruciferous veggies (bok choy, broccoli, brussels sprouts, cabbage, cauliflower), anything in the onion family (chives, garlic, leeks, onions, shallots), green leafies (collards, kale, spinach, dandelion greens), radishes, rutabaga, turnips
- **Fruits:** jicama, papaya, pineapple, tamarind
- **Grains:** bakery products, buckwheat, quinoa
- **Protein:** eggs, peanuts, tahini, soy products
- **Dairy:** all except pure butter, including goat and sheep milk products
- **Condiments and spices:** Carob and chocolate, horseradish, mustard, turmeric, yeast
- **Coffee**
- **Fermented foods:** miso, sauerkraut

Sulfur sensitivity goes back to one of two things: heavy metal toxicity, or a homozygous (two bad copies) genetic mutation in an enzyme called CBS (Cystathionine beta-synthase).

People with heavy metal toxicity can react strongly to sulfur containing foods because of the very strong affinity between sulfites and heavy metals: effectively, the sulfur-containing compounds can mobilize heavy metals. Anybody who has done IV heavy metal chelation can tell you that pulling a lot of metals out of the tissues at once can make you feel pretty lousy.

The CBS enzyme catalyzes (or drives) the recycling of sulfur containing compounds to get used for other things, releasing ammonia as a byproduct. Cysteine can then get incorporated back into glutathione. CBS mutations are usually up-regulations (meaning they work faster than normal), potentially resulting in an excess of sulfur-containing compounds, and also an excess of ammonia (symptoms of which include confusion, fatigue, weakness, poor appetite, nausea, and back or abdominal pain). These people already have too much sulfur; therefore, any food or supplement that adds to the pathway only worsens symptoms. (More on genetics and detoxification at the end of this chapter.)

Testing and Treatment for Sulfur Sensitivity

Your functional medicine doctor can usually tell if you are sensitive to sulfates based on results of an OAT test, or a routine homocysteine test (if it's low, it indicates this might be the issue). You can also find out if you have the CBS mutation via one of several genetic tests available online. The one I frequently use is called 23 & Me, taking their raw data and plugging it in to geneticgenie.org.

If you're high in sulfur or sulfites, you'll have to avoid high sulfur and thiol foods for a period of time—at least until your symptoms subside so that your sulfur-metabolizing enzymes can play catch-up. It's important to also avoid otherwise healthy sulfur-containing supplements, including ALA (Alpha Lipoic Acid), digestive enzymes derived from papaya and pineapple (bromelain and papain), chlorella, NAC (N-Acetyl Cysteine), DMSO, acidophilus if derived from dairy, glutathione, MSM (Methylsulfonylmethane), and turmeric.

The last step in eliminating sulfur from the body is an enzyme called sulfite oxidase, and it uses the mineral molybdenum as a cofactor. This can help.

Chlorophyll can help to neutralize excess ammonia. Since the dark leafy greens that contain chlorophyll also contain thiols, you can supplement with liquid chlorophyll.

Of course if you have an underlying heavy metal toxicity, gentle removal is the real treatment.

Toxic Personal Care Products

Skin care and beauty products often contain both the heavy metals and the endocrine disrupting chemicals (aluminum, fluoride, glycol ether) mentioned above. Unfortunately, topical products almost always contain at least some chemicals we don't recognize, even the so-called "clean" ones. That means you've got to read the labels very carefully!

Although many chemical ingredients have an identifiable name, it is worth mentioning that almost every product on the market contains **phthalates** (yes, the chemical previously mentioned in conjunction with soft plastics). The phthalates are not listed as such on the label though. They are hidden under the ingredient simply labeled "fragrance." You can bet that if the product is scented with anything other than natural essential oils, it will contain phthalates. For the rare product that is the exception, you can expect them to mention proudly on the label that it is phthalate-free. Phthalates were banned in the EU in plastic toys, but are still used in plenty of toiletry products.

Phthalates are not the only toxin in your scented products. About 95% of the chemicals used to make fragrances are derived from petroleum or benzene (the latter is very carcinogenic), and many of these are known toxins. They are linked to many allergic reactions and migraine cases, and patients who are chemically sensitive often cannot handle them at all. Again, avoid products listing "fragrance" on the ingredient list if you can.

Sodium Lauryl Sulphate or Sodium Laureth Sulfate (both called **SLS**) are found almost as frequently as phthalates and fragrances. Suspected carcinogens, SLS is linked to kidney and liver damage (and are associated with frequent UTIs), nervous system disruption, eye damage, eczema and dermatitis, and also linked with SLE (Lupus). They have been banned in Europe and Central America.

Only *slightly* less common that SLS in skin products, **propylene glycol** (found in antifreeze) is found in almost everything—even in many "natural" products, because it is FDA approved for food use. Propylene glycol, which has been banned in Europe, is toxic to the nervous system, clogs pores, and can actually speed up skin aging by depleting moisture from deeper skin layers.

Also found in many "natural" products are the **paraben** preservatives. Parabens mimic estrogens and are, unsurprisingly, associated with endocrine (hormonal) cancers. Specifically they have been linked with breast cancer. They are banned in Japan and Sweden, for obvious reasons. The ones you are most likely to encounter are **methylparaben** and **propylparaben**, but avoid any other words with a "-paraben" suffix also.

Case Study:

Peter grew up across the street from a farm, where chemical spraying occurred regularly. He had always been somewhat chemically sensitive, but it had worsened over time—most significantly after his mother passed away. He'd had some issues with GERD, or reflux, for years, but usually only after he went to bed. He'd managed it well enough until then with over the counter antacids. After his mom's death, though, he started to struggle with breakthrough reflux during the day, too. Around the same time, he began developing headaches in the presence of strong scents, such as perfumes or household cleaning supplies.

I told Peter that I suspected his liver had already been backed up, but stressors tend to decrease the body's ability to handle the resulting inflammation from an increased body burden (see Chapter 5). Basically, when you take an emotional hit, whatever your body's weak link is tends to blow!

We did IgG food allergy testing in that first visit, since reflux almost always goes back to food allergies. While we waited for those results to come back, I put him on a probiotic and DGL (deglycyrrhizinated licorice), a supplement to ease reflux symptoms, as well as NAG (N-Acetyl Glucosamine) to help heal the damage the reflux had caused so far. I also put Peter on a physical detox protocol involving sweating, alternating hot and cold, and castor oil packs (see the end of this chapter). I tried to convince him to do three colonics within the first two weeks, also, but those were a tough sell, particularly because he didn't have any constipation issues. So we decided to start with just the first three components of the protocol.

I also told him that while we were "emptying the trash bucket," he needed to be careful not to just keep piling more trash into his system at the same time. He already wasn't using commercial cleaning chemicals in his house, and his wife had long since given up scented personal care products due to his sensitivity. But we also discussed reading labels in both his food and his own personal care products. "If you don't recognize it, your liver won't either," I told him. We discussed doing genetic testing to optimize his liver's detoxification mechanisms, but he opted to hold off on that and try the rest of the protocol first.

Given the stress connection, I also recommended a salivary cortisol test to see how his adrenals were holding up (see Chapter 5). Peter admitted that he tended to be a "stuffer," keeping his emotions bottled up rather than processing and expressing them. I therefore also gave him a few referrals for grief counseling (he didn't seem interested in those), and a homeopathic remedy for suppressed grief. I told him the latter was often useful to help "open the door," as it were, to moving through the grief process so that it doesn't continue to cause physical problems. "If emotions come up when you take this, make sure you have a way to process them," I told him. "I'd also suggest you take it on a day when you don't have a lot of other things to do, just in case that does happen."

At Peter's first follow up, three weeks later, he told me (to his surprise) that his symptoms were already much improved. His reflux was well managed with the probiotics, the DGL and NAG, though he did still experience it every other day or so. He hadn't had any major emotional eruptions with the homeopathic remedy, but he did say he felt lighter and more hopeful from almost the first dose. With his wife's help, he'd also made great progress in eliminating all foreign chemicals from their food and his personal care products, and they'd even switched out all their plastic containers for glass.

At that first visit, based upon the results of testing, we put him on adrenal support and eliminated food allergies (he had quite a few), adding in glutamine to help heal up his gut lining over the next 6 weeks of avoidance.

Six weeks later, Peter said his reflux was completely gone, and he even forgot to take DGL and NAG most of the time. He'd sat behind a lady in church the previous week who wore a strong smelling perfume, and while he didn't enjoy it, he did not get a headache for the first time in years! Overall, his energy was better (he'd never even mentioned low energy to me before), and his mood had improved. He wanted to know how much longer he had to keep up with the physical detox protocol because it was "a pain." I told him it sounded like it had done its job for now, and he could stop, provided he continued to avoid those everyday chemicals that might increase his body burden once again. We also reintroduced those foods he had been sensitive to in a rotation fashion. We stopped the glutamine, though I told him to continue with the probiotics indefinitely.

As you can see from Peter's case, the daily burden of personal care chemicals were not in themselves the tipping point, but they contributed to a bigger picture. Once he'd done the work of cleaning up his liver, that allowed his gut to heal. It even allowed him to tolerate occasional chemical exposures without major symptoms.

Formaldehyde (aka formalin, formal and methyl aldehyde) is likewise banned in Japan and Sweden, but routinely used in the United States. Formaldehyde is used as a disinfectant and preservative, and it's a suspected carcinogen, especially linked with lung cancer. Exposure in high doses can cause asthma, headaches, eye irritation and upper respiratory irritation (I can attest to this firsthand from anatomy lab in medical school).

Anything ending in **-ethanolamine (Diethanolamine, Triethanolamine, Monoethanolamine)** should also be avoided. These chemicals are used as emulsifiers and foaming agents. Upon absorption, they become nitrosamines, which can cause cancer. They are also endocrine disruptors and skin irritants.

Toluene is a solvent toxic to the nervous system. It can also damage the liver, cause asthma, and disrupt the endocrine system. It is found mostly in nail-care products, but it is possible to find brands that are toluene-free.

Talc is also rather product specific: it is only found in powder products. Talc increases risk for ovarian cancer specifically, and for urinary tract infections when used in the genital area—so be sure, if you use powder, to choose a powder that is made from cornstarch. Talc is often found in cosmetic powder products, but there does not seem to be a direct link to toxicity from that route of exposure. I would try to avoid it if possible, especially if found in a loose face powder that may be inhaled.

Xylene (aka xytol or dimethylbenzene) is a surfactant (basically a cleanser) often found in cosmetics under the names **Ammonium Xylenesulfonate** and **Sodium Xylenesulfonate**. Xylene can damage your liver, and cause skin and respiratory tract irritation.

Over and over again, toothpaste in general ranks as highly toxic. Not only does toothpaste typically contain SLS, fluoride, artificial sweeteners, and propylene glycol, it often has DEA and Triclosan on the ingredient list as well. **Diethanolamine (DEA)** is used as an emulsifier and foaming agent, and upon absorption, it becomes a nitrosamine, which can cause cancer. It is also an endocrine disruptor. **Triclosan** is an antibiotic that has been associated with thyroid disruption. It also can form toxic byproducts when combined with the chlorine in water, such as carcinogenic dioxins.

All of this is a big deal, because chemicals that get absorbed through the mucosa in your mouth or through your skin don't go through what's called first pass metabolism, like the things you eat do. In first pass metabolism, what you eat stops at your liver for filtration before it's allowed into your bloodstream, but anything absorbed through your gums or your skin goes to the bloodstream directly.

When purchasing ready-made products, obviously it can be tough to avoid all of the toxic ingredients we just talked about. My general rule? Whenever possible I buy products with as few ingredients as possible—and I try to stick to those I recognize. If I just have to have a certain type of product, I scan the ingredient list for these primary offenders. If they aren't on there, I go ahead and buy it.

Does that mean there might still be something on the list that could cause some damage? Yep. But again, we live in a toxic world, and we can't control everything. I do the best I can and try not to obsess over the rest, since phobias are not healthy either!

Toxic Cleaning Products

Most companies that make personal care products deal in chemicals (the difference between "regular" and "natural" is only in the known toxicity of the ingredients); therefore, the company that makes your beauty products probably also makes your cleaning products. Those cleaning products are regulated even less stringently than are personal care products, and usually have a greater association with acute toxicity. The best thing to do is to read labels, and avoid those that come with a warning, such as "this could be fatal if inhaled," or "contact poison control immediately if X occurs," etc. Others may warn that the product may severely burn eyes and skin, may cause blindness or death, that the vapors are harmful or that you must use the product only while wearing gloves. Some labels even say things like "contain a substance known in (such-and-such state) to cause cancer," "probably carcinogenic to humans," or "prolonged exposure may cause reproductive and fetal effects." These are clues that *you do not want to buy that product.* (Do you want that stuff in your house, let alone in contact with your skin or lungs?)

It is also important to be careful of cleaning products with vague ingredients. Makers of cleaning products are not required to disclose their ingredients, and so many of them say things like "surfactant" or "solvent," without specifying their chemical nature. Personally, I wonder what they've got to hide… particularly because there are so many chemicals that have been linked with certain diseases, and some that have even been banned in other countries. If it all possible, I suggest that you avoid these products.

As far as actual ingredients, who's going to remember all those names? Even I have to look them up every time. My rule: if I don't recognize an ingredient, I don't buy it.

If everything you currently clean with breaks that rule, there are a number of green cleaning products available as alternatives—although you should read those labels as well, since some so-called green products are not as harmless as they claim. There are a few household staples that clean just about anything, though, so you shouldn't need to worry about specialty products too much. A non-toxic dish soap will clean just about any surface. (Really, try it.) If you need scrubbing power or odor elimination (those air fresheners and scented candles are poisonous![11]), add baking soda. This even works for ovens: Clean your oven by sprinkling baking soda liberally on the bottom. Spray with water, wait 8 hours, and then scrape and wipe the oven clean. And whatever dish soap and baking soda will not take care of can often be removed with vinegar. Vinegar cuts through grease, sanitizes counter tops (dilute to 50% if you have grout or other acid-sensitive surfaces), cleans windows, and even replaces fabric softener when added to your laundry's rinse cycle.

So, do your best with the natural cleaners and safer chemical products. But I must stress that it's not possible to completely avoid all harmful substances, and it's very possible to become obsessed with the attempt. That's not healthy either. My advice is to be educated, be wise, but try not to be fearful. Do what you can do, and let the rest go.

Toxins In Our Textiles

While I don't usually see textiles as a root cause of toxic body burden, it turns out that our wardrobes and linen closets can contribute to the overall toxic load. This can exacerbate inflammatory gut symptoms secondary to toxic overload.

Because of the way that our fibers are grown (or created) and the chemical treatments that are put onto the finished products, many of our fabric products are inherently toxic, and the way we care for those items often adds to the chemical burden inside of our homes.

Natural fibers such as cotton, linen, wool, cashmere, silk, and hemp are, in all, a better choice than synthetic fibers. But cotton is one of the top five pesticide-laden crops. Especially for things like pajamas (since you spend so much time in them), it may be worth it to track down organic cotton.

The manufacture of dyes for natural fibers often involves use of heavy metals such as cadmium, cobalt, and antimony. Thankfully, by choosing textiles colored with natural dyes, we can avoid yet another source of toxic metals.

Synthetic fabrics, such as acrylic, polyester, acetate, and nylon, are quite flammable, and therefore require additional chemical treatments (such halogenated flame retardants, or HFRs) to meet fire standards. HFRs have been linked to thyroid disruption, reproductive and developmental problems, immune suppression, and cancer.

Both natural and synthetic fabrics are routinely treated to be stain, static, or wrinkle resistant. This means they have added PFCs (perfluorochemicals). Your body cannot eliminate these easily, and they have been linked to reproductive and developmental toxicity, and cancers of the liver and bladder. Thankfully, most products in this category claim this on their tags, so it is not difficult to avoid them.

Aside from what is bonded into the textiles themselves, we release many toxins into our air from our laundering methods. You know now that many detergents have carcinogenic contaminants (unlabelled) and that you can use vinegar to replace those dryer sheets you can smell all the way outside. But perhaps you are not aware that dry cleaning is also a common source of solvent exposure.

Perchloroethylene, a volatile organic compound (VOC), is the most common dry cleaning agent. It absorbs into the clothing and does not wash out, and can enter the body through the lungs and skin. Long term exposure can cause liver and kidney damage, and causes cancer in animals. If you have items that must have specialty cleaning, eco-friendly dry cleaners use wet-cleaning technology and biodegradable detergents. If you can find one, they're a good alternative. Also, you may consider hand-washing some dry clean only items—often with natural fabrics, dry cleaning is not necessary, or may not be necessary after the first cleaning. The bottom line, though, is to avoid dry cleaning if you believe your gut inflammation might be secondary to a toxic burden. If you must dry-clean, hang the clothes in the garage to air out before bringing them inside, and consider wearing undergarments that limit the garment's contact with your skin.

It's not just the toxins in our clothing that can affect our health, but also the style. Constrictive fabrics limit lymphatic circulation (essentially recycled blood plasma). Your lymph is necessary for the immune system to remove waste, toxins, pathogens, and cancer cells. If circulation is inadequate, you can end up with fluid buildup in the tissues (edema), and limit the lymph system's necessary functions.

So be sure to wear clothes that you find comfortable and can move freely in. If you can find them made from untreated natural fibers, so much the better. And give yourself bonus points if they are naturally dyed!

A Word on Smoking

Cigarette smoke is another toxin that can contribute to the overall toxic load of the liver, filling up your "bucket" and spilling over into symptoms which can ultimately affect your gut. In addition to your toxic body burden, cigarette smoke is associated with a number of other serious diseases, including of course lung cancer, pancreatic cancer, cardiovascular disease (including strokes, aneurysms, and CHF), COPD, Alzheimer's Disease, and glaucoma—to name a few. Cigarette smoke contains a number of chemicals, many of which are carcinogenic. Here's a partial list:

- Benzene, also found in gasoline and a known carcinogen
- Polonium-210, which is radioactive and very toxic
- Vinyl Chloride, also used to make pipes
- Carbon monoxide, also found in car exhaust. It binds irreversibly with hemoglobin and prevents it from binding with oxygen.
- Hydrogen cyanide, used in chemical weapons
- Butane, used in lighter fluid
- Ammonia, used in household cleaners
- Toluene, used in paint thinners
- Cadmium, used in cigarette batteries, a known carcinogen

- Lead, once used in paint
- Arsenic, used in pesticides.

If you live with a smoker, encourage them to seek help with quitting (or at least ask them to smoke outside.) If you are the smoker, there are a few approaches that can help with quitting. Your Primary Care Physician may recommend nicotine-containing products that might work for you, such as gum, e-cigarettes, lozenges, patches, nasal sprays, and even a few oral meds that help modulate nicotine cravings. While these are not without their drawbacks, these alternatives are still preferable to smoking.

Alternatively, one of the most effective treatments I know for smoking cessation is auricular acupuncture. This is especially effective in conjunction with a taper down schedule for cigarettes, replacing them with a botanical or homeopathic combination to curb cravings. A basic healthy diet will also help to mitigate cravings, including avoiding sugar and processed foods, and getting some good nutrition.

Also, consider using peer pressure to your advantage. If you publicly announce that you plan to quit, it will (at least for most people) motivate you to stick with it—if the horrific list of possible smoking-affiliated ailments isn't enough.

Ways to Detox the Air in Your House

The air you breathe affects your overall body burden, too. Indoor air is typically two to five times more polluted than outdoor air. This is due to things like Volatile Organic Compounds (VOCs) from paint, furniture and flooring, as well as various toxic compounds in cleaning products, self-care products, dry cleaning products... you get the idea.

After tackling heavy metals, non-stick dishes, cleaning products, personal care products, textiles, and (if it applied to you) quitting smoking, your air should feel much fresher. But there are some extra steps you can take to really clean up what's left.

The easiest thing to do is to open a window (or two, or three), unless you have allergies to local pollens. This will at least dilute the polluted indoor air. If you need more air coming into your house, place a fan in front of the window, facing inside. If you are using something toxic, do the opposite and point the fan outside.

Because the bathroom air is even more polluted than the rest of the house, your bathroom should have an exhaust fan, and you should use it. If your bathroom has a window, so much the better—and you should definitely be running the fan and/or opening a window if you must use toxic cleaning or personal care products!

The same goes for your kitchen: if you have a vented range hood, use it. Bedrooms, on the other hand, don't have ventilation fans, but because you spend about a third of your life in your bedroom, you want to make sure it has really clean air.

Consider getting an air filter for your bedroom; High-Efficiency Particulate Air (HEPA) filters should be able to filter air up to 15 times per hour, and there are also air purifiers with carbon filters available if you still have a source of VOCs. (This is especially important if it's wintertime or cold much of the year where you live, and you can't open a window.) At the very least, if you must use cleaning products containing undisclosed or harmful chemicals for some reason, make sure you open a window, use a fan, or both.

Identifying a Toxic Liver

Let's revisit the trash bucket analogy: your liver is like your body's trash bucket. When you're born, it's empty (or at least it is for most of us). As you go through life, you encounter toxins, chemicals, organisms, and complex molecules that your body has to break down in order for them to be eliminated. These molecules get funneled into your "trash bucket"… and as long as it can keep up with the demand, you're okay. But as soon as the trash bucket gets too full, suddenly anything you try to throw into it spills out onto the floor (which in this case is your bloodstream). After that, even the most minor encounter with a substance that your liver would ordinarily need to process in order for elimination to occur will lead to symptoms. Very often, gut inflammation is one of those symptoms. There are five typical ways that this presents: chemical sensitivity, allergies, hormonal problems, and mold sensitivity.

You know your liver needs cleansing if you're really sensitive to chemicals. Patients with chemical sensitivities often say they have a major aversion to perfume, or cigarette smoke. Often they may have lived in a house under new construction (new materials tend to off-gas a lot), or worked in a building known to be toxic. Some will say they cannot handle using normal cleaning supplies, or even walking down the cleaning aisle at the store. Some have a hard time in big box stores (often cheaper clothing contains traces of formaldehyde). Some even swell up and develop itchy eyes or skin in the shower, as a reaction to the chlorine in tap water.

In addition to chemical sensitivity, it is pretty standard for liver toxicity to result in out-of-control allergies. Allergens are substances that are not inherently harmful to the body, but the body reacts as if they were harmful—the same way it might react to a pathogen. If the liver gets overwhelmed with toxins, either because of a massive exposure or because of cumulative exposures, some of those toxins will recirculate in the bloodstream. The immune system, thinking they are foreign invaders, will produce histamine. This is the reason why we suddenly develop seasonal allergies when the concentration of pollen in the air spikes, and the reason why some of us, as we get more "toxic," tend towards allergies all year round: you've suddenly exceeded your allergen threshold. (Note that high tendency towards allergies, especially food allergies, almost guarantees adrenal fatigue as well as liver toxicity.)

Our livers don't just filter toxins; they are also responsible for breaking down and eliminating our hormones. If your hormones are out of whack, it is a signal that your liver is too busy detoxing chemicals, or dealing with allergens. When chemicals and allergens get backed up, hormones get backed up too. This leads to recycling sex hormones, which can severely exacerbate or even cause PMS and menopausal symptoms in women.

Sensitivity to mold is both a cause of liver toxicity *and* a clue that the liver is toxic. Some molds produce mycotoxins (mold toxins) that are extremely poisonous to the body. This exposure typically happens through environmental exposure (most often in water damaged homes or buildings) or though food contamination. Because of the mycotoxins, some mold exposure can really clog up the liver, leading to all of these symptoms. I often see cases of inexplicable chemical sensitivities, allergies, and a host of physical symptoms all beginning with acute or severe exposure to mold.

If any of the above describes you, it is a sign that your liver may need some attention and a little assistance in doing its job.

Liver Cleansing Approaches

I tend to favor nutritional and (sometimes) mechanical approaches to liver cleansing over supplementation alone, as I often do not think supplements alone are strong enough to effect the quick change I'd like to see. Nutritional approaches include fasting in various forms, such as water and juice fasts, or guided medical food fasts. I use fasting as a sort of "reset button," decreasing overall inflammation in the body and allowing the liver and gut to flush out toxins. When the cleanse or fast is over, a clearer picture emerges of what still needs to be treated. If you fast, make sure you drink LOTS of water! This also helps your body to flush out toxins, much like rinsing out a bucket helps it get clean. Generally I recommend short juice fasts, no more than 3-5 days, and with a decreased schedule so that you don't end up fatigued. It's also important to check with your doctor before embarking on any kind of fast, as there are some people for whom this is not an appropriate choice—such as diabetics (juice fasting is very high in sugar), or those who are already weak or malnourished.

Detoxing Your Body

Because we live in a pretty toxic world, it's almost impossible to avoid at least some measure of regular exposure to chemicals, heavy metals, pesticides, and other offenders. While a major exposure resulting in a health crisis will require a full liver cleanse, it's a good idea to incorporate lighter detoxification rituals as often as you can.

We have discussed limiting your exposure to known toxins as much as you can by choosing your cleaning products, toiletry items, and food with care, but no matter how hard you try, you won't be able to avoid all toxic exposure. To keep toxic burden low on a regular basis, try incorporating some detox rituals into your daily or weekly routine.

An easy detoxification method to incorporate is dry brushing your skin before you shower. Even though it seems like this isn't doing much, dry skin brushing (from outer limbs towards the body's core) follows the line of lymphatic drainage. Your lymph is sort of a sewage system for toxins carried by your blood. Dry skin brushing helps to move toxins along so that they can reach some of the key elimination organs to be eliminated.

Another detoxification ritual is to make sure you sweat on a regular basis. Many toxins are fat-soluble, and sweat helps liberate them from the fat cells and usher them into the bloodstream, where they will eventually find their way to the liver, and, if all works well, into the gut and out of the body.

You can support your liver in removing those toxins by eating more cruciferous veggies. Cruciferous veggies are the ones that "flower outward"—like broccoli, cauliflower, bok choy, and brussels sprouts. These vegetables are all great sources of sulfur, which is required for three of the liver's Phase II detoxification pathways.

Eating plenty of fermented foods supports the next stop in the toxin removal pathway: your gut. Fermented foods are packed with probiotics, which are extremely important for your digestive health. An integral part of the raw diet, these used to be a much bigger component of our diets than they are today. (One caveat to this: if you think you might have candida overgrowth, or SIBO, you'll want to hold off on fermented foods until you fully address those problems. More on this in Chapter 4.)

If you want to liberate even more stored toxins, try juicing your veggies. I don't always recommend juicing over eating the veggies whole, particularly if you have insulin resistance, candida overgrowth, or sugar addiction, because juicing removes the fiber and leaves the sugar. But it also leaves the nutrients, and does not require much effort on the part of your digestive system in order to absorb them. This makes fresh juices perfect for cleansing purposes.

A Little Help for the Detox Process

Before beginning this process, please make sure you check with your health care provider to make sure this is appropriate for you. Some very sensitive patients cannot handle even this gentle detoxification approach.

To really kickstart your whole-body cleanse, for many people I recommend a series of four steps: sauna or sweating, alternating hot and cold (otherwise known as constitutional hydrotherapy), castor oil packs, and colonics. This is because the body has a couple of natural methods of eliminating toxins. In naturopathic theory, we call them "emunctories," and they are your breath, sweat, urine, and bowel movements. When the body is functioning optimally, the emunctories are open, and toxins are easily eliminated. However, one of the causes of disease involves clogging these routes of elimination, leading to toxic buildup, and eventually dysfunction. Any one of these emunctories can be blocked. Following the protocol listed above is sort of like squeezing a tube of toothpaste from the bottom: the sauna or sweating releases fat-soluble toxins from adipose tissue into the bloodstream; hydrotherapy flushes the blood to the liver; castor oil packs cause the liver to "dump" into the colon, and colonics help to flush the toxins out of the body. Let's take them one at a time.

Sauna

In addition to detoxification, spending time in the sauna has several other health benefits: if done after a workout, it increases recovery and muscle relaxation, it brings more blood flow to the skin's surface, it's good for your heart (almost a cardiovascular workout in itself!), it increases the production of white blood cells, and it improves sleep quality. If you belong to a gym with a sauna, tack on a session at the end of your workout whenever you can. If you don't, you can still get many of these benefits just by making sure you work out to a sweat.

Hydrotherapy

Hydrotherapy dates back to the 1800s, when a priest named Father Kneipp first began to use the properties of hot and cold water applications to heal. There are really only two basic principles involved in all forms of hydrotherapy. The first principle is that hot applications (of any kind, water included) cause vasodilation (they make your blood vessels expand), while cold applications cause your blood vessels to constrict. The second principle is that there are two responses of your body to any stimulus: the first, or primary action, and the secondary, lasting action. Any living system is designed to maintain homeostasis, or balance, and so both actions are always necessary. For instance, if you ice your injured shoulder, then the primary response is that the local blood vessels will constrict and decrease the flow of blood (and thus decrease inflammation). But after awhile, your body realizes that if it wants to prevent frostbite, it had better send some blood to that shoulder—so the secondary response is an increased blood flow to the area. The same happens with heat: the primary effect is vasodilation, but the secondary effect is decreased blood flow to the surface.

These principles can be applied in a variety of ways, depending on the condition. In constitutional hydrotherapy, which I recommend for detoxing, it involves a series of alternating hot and cold towels to the torso. These create a sort of "pumping" action, bringing blood to the internal organs and then flushing it away quicker than would otherwise occur physiologically. This increases the flow of oxygen and nutrients, and whisks away toxins faster as well. Water is an especially good vehicle for this effect, because it has a high specific heat, which allows it to absorb and give off large quantities of heat. If you can find a medical spa that offers this treatment, wonderful; if you can't, you can simulate it in your home, or just alternate between hot and cold in the shower. I recommend three cycles, about a minute each: start on hot, and end cold. If you're not chlorine sensitive and you belong to a gym, you can also alternate between the hot tub and the pool after sitting in the sauna.

Castor Oil Packs

Castor oil penetrates the skin well, causing a local "inflammatory" reaction—in a good way. It alerts the body to bring more blood flow to the area, which means more oxygen and nutrients, and faster waste elimination, triggering the liver to "dump" into the colon. To apply a castor oil pack, pour cold pressed castor oil on a flannel sheet, folded to fit the area of treatment (in this case, over your liver: underneath the right side of your ribcage). Then apply the saturated sheet to treatment area, and cover with saran wrap to hold the flannel sheet in place and protect your clothing. (You can skip the saran wrap, but then you won't be able to move around much during treatment.) Next, apply a heating pad on top of the flannel sheet, and relax for 20-30 minutes.

Colonics

Finally, colonics can help with toxic elimination in two ways. The first is obvious: colonic irrigation manually cleans out the bowels, which may be necessary from time to time for people who suffer from chronic constipation.

The second way that colonics can help with detoxification has to do with bile dumping. Bile is produced by the liver, stored by the gall bladder, and secreted in response to the ingestion of fatty foods. Because fat does not readily mix with the water contents of the gut, it requires emulsification with bile salts in order to absorb the calories and nutrients. However, bile also absorbs fat-soluble toxins for the same reason it absorbs fatty foods. When this happens, it is important to be able to eliminate these toxins.

Even in healthy individuals, a high percentage of the body's bile is reabsorbed in the terminal ileum (the last part of the small intestine), which means all of the remaining fat-soluble toxins get recirculated into the bloodstream. In constipated individuals, the percentage of reabsorbed bile approaches 90-95%. Although colonics only reach the colon and not the small intestine, they have nevertheless been shown to increase the dumping of bile, thereby decreasing the recirculation of fat-soluble toxins.

I'd repeat the first three steps about 3-4 times per week for at least 6 weeks. In general, I recommend a series of three colonics over a two week period at the beginning of your cleanse. After that, just make sure you're having good, substantial bowel movements daily.

Genetics: A *Lot* of Help for the Detox Process

All of this works great, as long as your liver is reasonably good at its job. Unfortunately, some of us have SNPs, or Single-Nucleotide Polymorphisms, in the genes encoding certain enzymes necessary in the liver's detoxification process.

Quick genetics interlude: for every gene, you get two copies, one from your mother and one from your father. If you get two "good" (i.e. functional) copies of a given gene, all is well. If you get one "good" and one "bad" copy, you have what's called a heterozygous mutation (*hetero-* means different than). If you're otherwise healthy, the good copy can compensate for the bad copy, and you're still all right, as long as you take good care of yourself.

But if you get two "bad" copies, you have a homozygous mutation (*homo-* means same as). These are the ones that can significantly impair your liver's ability to eliminate toxins. SNPs that often contribute to liver detoxification impairment are MTHFR, NAT1, NAT2, GSTM1, CBS, and PON1. There are a number of labs now that will test your genetics and give you this information; many of them will also test quite a few of your cytochrome systems (all of which begin with CYP- and have a series of numbers after them. Cytochrome systems are specific to certain types of chemicals or drugs, and will only affect those.)

While it's not possible to change your genetics (at least at the time of this writing!), what you can do is optimize the function of the enzymes those genes encode for by giving them the vitamin and mineral cofactors they need. This will enable those enzymes, impaired though they are, to work as efficiently as possible. I'd recommend finding a functional medicine or naturopathic physician to help you with this process if you suspect you have this problem.

The Take-Home Message:

- **Buy personal care products containing only a short list of ingredients.**
- **If you don't recognize the ingredient, don't put it on your body.**
- **Buy natural fabrics** whenever possible.
- **Open your windows** whenever possible.
- **Consider purchasing a HEPA filter** for rooms where you spend the bulk of your time.
- Incorporate **dry skin brushing** into your daily or weekly routine, perhaps before a shower.
- If you know that you are toxic, **consider committing to at least six weeks** of sauna, hydrotherapy, castor oil packs, and a series of colonics at the beginning.
- If you're really toxic, see a naturopathic or functional medicine doctor to help you support your genetic detoxification mechanisms.

Chapter

3

BIOTOXINS AND CHRONIC INFECTIONS = GUT INFLAMMATION

B
iotoxins are a very common obstacle to cure for guts that just won't heal—particularly candida or yeast overgrowth that simply won't stay gone despite what would otherwise be more than adequate treatment, or food allergies that return with a vengeance even after avoidance of allergens and appropriate gut healing nutrients. When I see these kinds of cases, I start looking for deeper obstacles to cure. Often, the cause turns out to be biotoxins. (If your quiz from the introduction did not imply that this chapter was for you, though, I invite you to skip to Chapter 4!)

The two most common biotoxin illnesses I see are Lyme Disease and toxic mold. In many cases, they go together. Lyme is a spirochete bacteria that comes from (usually) a tick bite, though there are other organisms that can transfer it too. Toxic mold comes from exposure to a water damaged building. You wouldn't expect there to be any relationship between these two scenarios... and at least according to the CDC, Lyme should be quite rare (though from what I've seen, it's very under-diagnosed.) So why do these two illnesses so often coexist?

Unfortunately I haven't been able to find a definitive answer—the experts seem to agree that they *do* go together, but the closest I've found to a possible explanation is that the biotoxins from one increase the immune system's susceptibility to the biotoxins of the other.

With that in mind, here's what we do know.

TGFb1: A Marker for Biotoxins

The TGFb1 blood test is a marker for biotoxins from one of two sources: toxic mold, or Lyme.[2] Because it only spikes from one or the other, my next step is typically to run a Lyme Western Blot. If Lyme is as under-diagnosed as I think it is, then it might just be an incidental finding: we find it because we're looking for it, and it's more prevalent than we think it is.

HLA DR: A Genetic Test for Post-Lyme Syndrome, Mold Biotoxin Illness, or Both

The HLA DR blood test helps determine whether a patient is genetically susceptible to toxic mold[2] (about a quarter of the population is), and it also happens to test for whether a patient is susceptible to Post-Lyme Syndrome— or lingering fatigue, gut dysfunction, joint pain or muscle aches even after Lyme is gone. According to the CDC, the cause of Post-Lyme Syndrome is not known.[3] My suspicion, since these are all biotoxin-related illnesses and Lyme does produce neurotoxins, is that Post-Lyme Syndrome is a result of the body's inability to detoxify Lyme neurotoxins. According to some Lyme literate doctors, Post-Lyme Syndrome is actually a lingering Lyme infection, though.

So again: susceptibility to biotoxins often overlaps, regardless of the source.

Detoxification Problems

I have yet to see a toxic mold patient who is not also sensitive to everyday household chemicals such as perfumes, cleaning agents, detergents, and the like. Most of them also have increased intestinal permeability, or "leaky gut syndrome": that is, they're sensitive to lots of different foods (see Chapter 1). I often see this in Lyme patients, as well. Here's why.

Back to the trash bucket analogy: if your liver is a big trash bucket, biotoxins (from mold and Lyme both) have to get processed by your liver, too—and in the sicker patients, there are a lot of them (indirectly measured by either TGFb1, c3a, or c4a). This means the bucket fills up faster.

But it's also possible (and common, from what I've seen) for patients susceptible to biotoxin illnesses to also have less efficient liver detoxification mechanisms in the first place. (To continue the analogy, they have smaller trash buckets.) This can be measured with genetic testing of SNPs (mutations) in the liver's various cytochrome enzymes, as mentioned at the end of Chapter 2. Again, while genes can't be fixed (yet), we can at least optimize their function by giving the less efficient enzymes the vitamins and minerals they need to work as well as they can.

I don't think this explains the connection between mold and Lyme, but it does at least in part explain why the symptom pictures between the two often look so similar. Another possibility is that Lyme appears to be an opportunist—that is, not everyone who is exposed to it develops symptoms. In those individuals, symptom development requires a priming event which weakens the immune system—such as mold exposure.

If you have a biotoxin-induced illness, even if you know you were exposed to a water-damaged building and that is likely the cause, I'd recommend getting checked for Lyme Disease anyway. (This requires a Western Blot, and chances are quite high that it will be officially negative—but the bands present will give away whether you have been exposed to Lyme or not. This, combined with a CD-57 test and the symptom picture, will usually determine whether or not Lyme is a current contributing factor to your illness.)

While you're at it, check your HLA-DR. If you have a clear biotoxin illness and you're genetically susceptible to either mold or Lyme but not the other, that can help point you in a clear clinical direction.

So much for biotoxin illnesses in general—now let's look at each of them in turn.

Mold Toxicity

When I first started seeing the test results for toxic mold in my practice I was incredulous. Why were so many people showing up in my office with mold sickness—in bone-dry Tucson, Arizona, of all places?

It turns out that, while mold grows in damp places, spores can survive in incredibly adverse conditions,[4] including in dry deserts—and reanimate when the conditions are better. Like in your walls after a rain (particularly if you have drywall). Or in your vents. Or under your sink. Or in your floorboards after a leak.

What Mold Is

There are three primary categories of microorganisms involved in human illness (not counting the parasites): viruses, bacteria, and fungi. Mold is in the third category.

Most of us think of mold as the black stuff we can see, but fungi release spores into the air to reproduce. Sometimes this can give off a musty smell, but sometimes if you're not sensitive, you won't see or smell a thing. That's part of what can make mold so tricky to diagnose. It can also grow almost anywhere there's dampness and oxygen.

Types of Mold

- **Allergenic mold**: These don't usually cause problems unless you're allergic and/or exposed to a lot of them. These include alternaria, cladosporium, and penicillum.
- **Pathogenic mold**: These are molds that can produce infections if you're immunocompromised. Aspergillus is one example, as it can cause the lung infection aspergillosis. There seem to be a number of people with an unspecified toxic, pathogenic mold inhabiting their sinus cavities. In some cases they may present with a fungal ball visible on imaging tests but, more often than not, testing is unreliable. There are a few doctors that have had success treating such infections with long-term use of prescription antifungals, often intranasal for sinus infections.

- **Toxic mold**: These molds release mycotoxins and are harmful regardless of allergic potential. Aspergillus also releases mycotoxins so it would fit here too, as do some species of penicillum (this is where we get the antibiotic penicillin from). The most toxic form of mold is stachybotrys, or "black mold." You can absorb the mycotoxin produced by stachybotrys, trichothecenes, through your gut, lungs, and skin. It is fat-soluble, so you can also store it for a long time.

Screening for Mold

Some of my patients will get swab test kits (like from moldscreeningkit.com for $100 at the time of this writing) or petri dishes from Home Depot, and I believe they run around $30. But these only work for mold you can see (which is useful, because it's possible to mistake allergenic molds for stachybotrys, and the only way to know what you've got for sure is to test it). If you suspect mold but can't see it, the best way to find out if you have a problem is with an ERMI test. You can purchase one here: https://www.mycometrics.com/products.html. The ERMI score should come back less than 2 in order to indicate safety. HERTSMI-2 tests are useful after remediation has been completed, to make sure that mold is no longer present.

It's possible to test for antibodies against some of the types of mold listed, but this will only tell you if you are allergic; it won't tell you if you're toxic from mold exposure. The best test for this is the cytokine TGFb1. Others that can help inform it are complement c3a and c4a, and MSH.[2] If your test results show exposure to biotoxins and you have a mold-sensitive HLA-DR *or* your Western Blot is completely negative, you almost certainly have mold toxicity.

I've also run a specialty test in some cases that measures mycotoxins directly, but I do this rarely and usually upon request, as it is pricey.

Case Study:

Valerie was a 21 year old college student who came to me with chronic diarrhea and weight loss, as well as abdominal pain, joint pain in her low back and her hips, and insomnia. She had already been to see a gastroenterologist and a rheumatologist before coming to me, ruling out any traditional causes of malabsorption syndrome or autoimmunity. When asked when the symptoms started, she said two years ago, after a trip to Mexico. We wondered about parasites.

I flipped towards the back of the new patient paperwork, and saw that she had marked sensitivity to most household chemicals, and had checked the box next to "lived or worked in a toxic or moldy environment."

"When was that?" I asked her.

Valerie thought of a minute, and then said, "about two years ago. When I got back from Mexico. I don't live there anymore though—I moved out about six months ago."

A-ha, I thought. "So there are two possible causes here, and maybe they both apply, but we won't know until we do a little more testing," I said. "If your house had toxic mold in it, that certainly could cause systemic inflammation and liver backup, which is the likely cause of all your chemical sensitivities. I've also seen mold as the underlying cause to leaky gut syndrome plenty of times before, which can lead to malabsorption too. If you're one of the quarter of the population that is genetically sensitive to toxic mold, it might still be affecting you even now. Of course, it's also possible you were exposed to a parasite, so we should check for that too."

We did food allergy testing, in order to remove the inflammatory insults preventing the gut from healing, and since I knew I'd be putting her on glutamine and probiotics regardless of the results, we did that right away. We also ran a comprehensive stool culture, to identify not only parasites, but good and bad bacteria balance, yeast overgrowth, markers for inflammation that might indicate Irritable Bowel Disease, markers for occult blood, and much more. I also sent her to test a common marker indicating the presence of mold biotoxins, TGFb1.

For some immediate relief from fatigue and support for her inflammatory symptoms, I put her on Adrenal Support. We opted not to run a salivary cortisol test that first visit, since we were running several other specialty tests, and wanted to keep costs down.

"Let's cut out the foods you're sensitive to and combine the elimination diet with a candida protocol for the yeast," I said. The stool culture also tested sensitivity of her bacteria to various natural and prescription medications, so we added in Grapefruit Seed Extract to kill off the dysbiotic bacteria. "Secretory IgA will continue to increase with glutamine and as we eliminate the food allergies," I added.

"What about this?" Valerie asked, pointing at the TGFb1 number.

"Mold biotoxins can be eliminated from the body using an off-label cholesterol medication called cholestyramine," I told her. "It's a binder, and it has no systemic effects: in the gut, it binds cholesterol and pulls it out of the body. It does the same thing to mold biotoxins. All else being equal, the cholestyramine should drop the TGFb1 by about 2000 points per month, in my experience; given your level, that means you'll likely need to be on it for about six months." Valerie blinked at me, wide-eyed and shaking her head. "How did this happen?" She sounded a little overwhelmed.

"Well, my suspicion was that the trip to Mexico led to the bacterial contamination, and the mold exposure made a bad situation much worse. Both led to inflammation and leaky gut, and that led to overgrowth of yeast. But the good news is, now we know the problems, and we can treat them."

At her next follow up six weeks later, Valerie was thrilled. Her diarrhea had stopped, the abdominal pain was gone, and her joint pain had vanished. She was also sleeping well, her energy had improved, and best of all, she'd gained eight pounds.

"Great!" I told her. "I would stay off of sugar and more or less stay on the candida diet plan until the TGFb1 markers are in normal range, or else the organism is likely to grow back; mold is a common obstacle to cure for that. I'd also continue to avoid the foods with the highest sensitivity titers, but you can add the others back in a rotation fashion."

We continued to monitor her for the next few months to make sure the TGFb1 numbers continued to decrease, and at last we were able to get her off of cholestyramine. She even went back to having sugar and desserts occasionally, with no problems.

Mold Treatment

Mold treatment usually involves remediation and/or avoidance, binding and eliminating it (with activated charcoal, or prescription medications cholestyramine[4] or colestipol), and treating the other fungi that tend to come with it (usually candida or other yeast). Sometimes a good detox protocol is also necessary, especially for patients who also have a lot of chemical sensitivities in addition to mold issues. Leaky gut also shows up secondary to this more often than not.

Some cases clear up pretty quickly after getting away from the mold source, and some are more complicated. But definitely the first step is finding out whether mold is part of your issue.

Case Study:

Helen developed reflux after going to work for a company whose building I suspected of toxic mold, having seen several of their employees already. She started taking a PPI (proton pump inhibitor), after which she also developed atrophic gastritis, nausea, and severe fatigue.

I told her that I suspected the PPI caused the gastritis, and the reflux was probably a result of food allergies due to leaky gut syndrome, secondary to mold exposure. We confirmed this with food allergy testing, treated the mold with cholestyramine, and started a cocktail of supplements to help heal up her gastritis. She also came back positive for candida antibodies—not surprising, since candida and mold nearly always go together. We put her on a candida protocol and eliminated food allergies too.

Six weeks later, her energy was much improved, her reflux was mostly gone, and her nausea was gone. We were able to taper her off the PPI over a several month period after that with no problems. Unfortunately she continued to work in the moldy environment for another few years, so she had to stay on the cholestyramine until she was able to find other employment.

Lyme Disease

If you have a biotoxin illness but all the tests for mold exposure are normal, it is likely that you will be positive for Lyme disease.

Lyme disease is a tick-borne bacterial illness most commonly associated with outdoor activities in New England. It was first reported in Connecticut in 1975, but unfortunately, it didn't stay where it came from. Although there is still a higher prevalence of Lyme in the New England states than in, say, Arizona, it is far from unheard of here. But because it can look like so many other conditions, it often goes undiagnosed.

Lyme is transmitted via tick bite, and the infection at first is local. Classically, Lyme presents with a "bullseye" rash (also known as *erythema migrans*) near the bite location, though many patients later confirmed to carry the bacteria responsible for Lyme (called *Borrelia burgdorferi*) recall neither a tick nor a rash. Other early non-specific symptoms can be mistaken for a flu-like illness. These symptoms may include chills, fever, malaise, headache, muscle pain, stiff neck, and sometimes lightheadedness and itching. If the illness is caught at this stage, four weeks of antibiotic therapy should get rid of it.

If it is not caught, Lyme usually disseminates throughout the body weeks to months later, affecting the joints and the nervous system. Common chronic Lyme includes neurological symptoms like tingling and numbness, vision changes, light and sound sensitivity, speech disturbances, and nerve pain. Other common symptoms include cognitive deficits ("brain fog"), fatigue, palpitations, and joint pain. Most of my Lyme patients also experience chronic gut inflammation, food reactions, and occasionally abdominal cramping. A fair number of them may also have had mold exposure; these go together fairly frequently.

Case Study:

Janette came to me with bloating and severe allergies, especially seasonal allergies, which worsened when she came to Arizona years earlier. She removed her IgE food allergens and did immunotherapy to desensitize her to the local flora and fauna, but she continued to struggle. As we chatted, she also said both bloating and allergies got much better when she avoided gluten and dairy. Then she mentioned a history of mold exposure—at which point I was no longer sure if gluten and dairy avoidance helped her because of an allergy to those foods, or due to candida overgrowth, since candida tends to go along with mold biotoxins.

We tested her for TGFb1, and it was quite high, as were candida antibodies. We also did food allergy testing (IgG), showing leaky gut syndrome. I told her that I suspected the mold was the underlying cause of both her leaky gut syndrome and the yeast overgrowth. I put her on cholestyramine anyway, but just to rule it out, I also sent her to check for Lyme Disease too.

At her one month follow-up, cholestyramine had dropped the TGFb1 number dramatically, suggestive that mold really had been the cause of its elevation… but her HLA DR showed that she was susceptible to post-Lyme syndrome, and she was also positive for Lyme. My suspicion was that her mold exposure triggered the latent bacteria to come out of its "resting" phase.

Since she was feeling so much better and we'd already worked at cleaning up her body's "terrain," this was the perfect time to treat Lyme with minimal risk of die-off, or Herxheimer reactions. We put her on the herbal protocol by Stephen Buhner. As expected, she tolerated them quite well.

Her bloating is now gone, and as long as she minimizes the foods on her "sensitive" list, she can eat them occasionally without a problem.

Testing for Lyme Disease

Testing for Lyme can be tricky. First, Borrelia doesn't even trigger a rise in even the body's initial antibodies (IgM) until 4-6 weeks after infection. These IgM antibodies later convert to IgG antibodies several months down the line. You have to test at precisely the right time to catch them.

Second, Borrelia IgG fades over time—not because the infection is gone, but because Borrelia learns to evade the immune system. This means the Western Blot (a lab test which identifies proteins in a tissue sample by molecular weight) is almost always negative—though Lyme-specific bands will give away whether or not a patient has been exposed. Therefore it's usually necessary to run a CD57, suppressed in chronic Lyme. I've also started running complement c3a and c4a in addition, as I've found c4a tends to spike more often with mold, and c3a more often with Lyme (though they can both elevate with either).

Another complication: often, ticks infected with Lyme carry other organisms as well, including Babesia, Bartonella, Ehrlichia, mycoplasma, and others. On top of that, lowered immune function accompanying all this often allows chronic viruses to flare, including Epstein Barr, Human Herpes Virus 6, and Cytomegalovirus, as well as fungal infections like candida.

Treating Lyme

Before anything else, I always start by treating yeast overgrowth, nutritional, or hormonal deficiencies. This approach makes treatment of Lyme and coinfections easier and more effective.

Often, during treatment of Lyme and coinfections, it's necessary to also treat biofilms. These are aggregates of organisms that adhere to each other and to a body surface, covering themselves with a layer of DNA, proteins, sugars, and fats to protect themselves from discovery by the immune system. It's hard to test for biofilms, so more often than not, I just assume they're present and treat them, using natural products like enzymes and Grapefruit Seed Extract. This allows either the antibiotics or the herbs (depending on the treatment approach chosen) to penetrate and treat the infection.

One more complication: Borrelia has multiple configurations: the L-form, which hides inside cells, the more traditional spiral form, and the cystic form. If I treat with antibiotics, I'll often pulse dose with different types in an effort to treat all three. The herbal approach is more of a long, steady process.

Throughout the protocol, we support the patient's detoxification pathways to minimize "die-off," or Herxheimer reactions: as organisms die, fragments spill into the bloodstream, triggering immune responses and flu-like symptoms.

Supporting detoxification (and adding binders, like activated charcoal, to grab the fragments and pull them out of circulation) helps minimize die-off discomfort.

Treatment takes (minimum) two months on the antibiotics, though it is usually longer. On the herbs, it can be much longer: generally eight to twelve months. If you combine the two, it might be somewhere in between. When symptoms subside, we start checking CD57 to make sure it's coming up, as well as TGFb1.

Chronic Viral Infections

Chronic viral infections occurring on their own don't usually present with gut symptoms... but they do often show up along with biotoxin illnesses, and biotoxin illnesses generally *do* cause gut symptoms. Viral infections need to be addressed as well, in order for the illness to fully heal.

Viruses work by using your own cellular machinery against you. They latch on to the cell membrane, insert their DNA (or RNA) into the cell, and convince the cell to manufacture its proteins for it.

A strong and healthy immune system can fight off and eradicate most viral infections, but certain viruses never completely disappear. This is because they hide out in your cells, dormant, waiting to be reactivated... and your immune system won't know to attack because from the outside, nothing abnormal is going on. Viruses in the Herpes family (Epstein Barr Virus, Human Herpes Virus 6, Herpes Simplex 1 and 2, and Cytomegalovirus) fall under this category. These viruses are opportunists, which means they reactivate whenever the immune system is down for the count because it's too busy dealing with something else.

When you first get infected with a virus, your body makes an immunoglobulin called IgM specific to that virus to fight it off. These stay elevated only for the first 6-12 weeks; so if you suspect the infection is that new, this would be the one to look for.

After that period of time, the IgM numbers (think of these as your first line of defense) will die down to zero, and instead you'll have elevated IgG (think of these as the reserves). These can tell you that you either have an active chronic infection, or that you had a past infection and the reserves are sticking around to make sure nobody gets out of hand again.

There isn't really a definitive way to tell whether the elevated IgG numbers are due to an active or a past infection unfortunately. Typically I look for titer numbers: very high antibody counts suggest that active recruitment is still happening because the invaders aren't gone. You can also check for the DNA of the invader; high DNA material indicates that the virus is replicating. Lower titers imply a past infection.

While there are some prescription antiviral therapies that can be effective, a few natural treatments that are effective include:

Mycelial extracts from mushrooms: these can be more effective than many antiviral drugs.

Coconut oil (or its powerful antiviral extract, Monolaurin)

Lysine: this is an amino acid that prevents replication of HSV 1 and 2 by inserting itself in place of an amino acid these viruses do require (arginine). It's not known for certain whether it will do the same for all the other viruses in the Herpes family, but I've used it with good clinical results.

The Take-Home Message:

If you suffer from mysterious symptoms in addition to digestive disturbances, struggle with chronic fatigue or sensitivity to multiple chemicals, consider asking your doctor to evaluate you for biotoxin illnesses and chronic infections. These might be your obstacle to cure.

Chapter
4

DYSBIOSIS AND CANDIDA

D ysbiosis is a general term for overgrowth of opportunistic or pathogenic gut flora. Usually it refers to bacterial overgrowth, though it does also encompass candidiasis, or overgrowth of the form of yeast known as candida. Either or both can occur on their own, or secondary to other gut pathologies, such as leaky gut syndrome (see Chapter 1).

Not every possible cause of dysbiosis will apply to you in this section. In order to help you skip to the sections most relevant to your case, I recommend that you first take the following quiz to help you navigate to the sections most relevant to you.

What are Your Most Likely Causes of Dysbiosis?
1. Do you feel worse when you eat carbs (sugar, bread, pasta, etc)? Y/N
2. Do probiotics often make you feel worse? Y/N
3. Do you feel worse when you eat fruit sugar (fructose), garlic, onions, legumes, and sugar alcohols like erythritol or sorbitol or maltitol? Y/N

4. Do you have a history of autoimmunity, such as Hashimoto's, Lupus, Rheumatoid Arthritis, etc? Y/N
5. Do you have any blood or mucus in your stool? Y/N
6. Do your symptoms flare when you eat nuts and seeds, chocolate, wine, cheese, avocados, and/or fermented foods? Y/N
7. If you are a woman, have you ever used birth control pills? Y/N
8. Have you ever used many rounds of antibiotics, or had a round recently, particularly of one like Keflex? Y/N
9. Have you used any acid blocking medications, such as omeprazole or Dexilant? Y/N

Key:

If yes to 1-2, read the SIBO section

If yes to 3: read the FODMAPs section

If yes to 4: read the Autoimmune Protocol section, and also make sure you read chapters 1-3, depending on which of them applied best in your quiz from the introduction!

If yes to 5: read the Specific Carbohydrate section

If yes to 6: read the Histamine Intolerance section

If yes to 7: read the Birth Control Pills section and the Candidiasis section

If yes to 8: read the Antibiotics and the Candidiasis sections

If yes to 9: read the PPI and the Candidiasis sections.

Candidiasis

Candidiasis, or candida albicans overgrowth, happens because your gut has its own microscopic ecosystem that needs to stay in balance. Everyone has a trace amount of candida in their guts—but these little guys are opportunists. That means that they don't play offense, but as soon as the good bacteria get wiped out (by a hefty round of antibiotics, say), they will proliferate and fill in the empty space. Nature abhors a vacuum (so said Aristotle).

Candida is a single-celled fungus, or a yeast, and it eats sugar. I tend to think of this when people tell me they're addicted to sugar, or when a diet diary shows me they're eating either a lot of sugar or white carbs (which are essentially the same thing).

Because candida eats sugar, people with candidiasis crave it. In a vicious cycle, they'll eat lots of sugar, triggering the pancreas to release a bolus of insulin to reduce glucose levels that would otherwise be toxic. Then sugar rushes out of the bloodstream and into the cells, and blood sugar crashes. This leads to shakes and irritability, a condition called hypoglycemia—and even more sugar cravings.

As a byproduct of its sugar metabolism, candida produces acetaldehyde, the same toxic byproduct your liver produces when processing alcohol. (Acetaldehyde is actually the chemical responsible for hangovers.) So effectively, candida can make you feel a little bit drunk. People usually describe it as poor memory, fuzzy thinking, or poor word recall. Acetaldehyde can also lead to headaches.

Because candida ferments the sugar you eat, you can end up with gas and bloating. One of the byproducts of fermentation is carbon dioxide which, as you can probably imagine, is great in your lungs, but pretty unpleasant in your gut.

Sometimes, when candida overgrowth gets really out of hand, a patient will have yeast issues on their skin. You may recognize this as jock itch, vaginitis, athlete's foot, ringworm, intertrigo, or thrush. Sometimes, though, a patient will end up itching at some other body orifice, often the ears, the anus, or the throat.

When candida overgrowth gets out of control, it ends up irritating the gut lining, and over time this can cause inflammation. If the inflammation is severe enough, it can lead to food molecules prematurely coming in contact with the bloodstream, and this can trick your body into thinking the food is a foreign invader. This is intestinal hyperpermeability, or "leaky gut syndrome" (see Chapter 1). It causes food allergies and sensitivities, and can complicate treatment. It is also possible for the inflammation from intestinal hyperpermeability to cause dysbiosis: the two conditions are mutually reinforcing.

To effectively treat candida, you need to 1) identify and remove the obstacle to cure (which may be a high sugar diet, tapering off a PPI or birth control pill, or remediating a moldy house), 2) starve it by restricting what it eats (eliminate white carbs, sugar and yeast) for either six weeks, or as long as it takes for you to remove the obstacle to cure, 3) kill it using either natural or prescription antifungals, and 4) repopulate with the good stuff (probiotics).

For personalized help with this process, I recommend seeing a functional medicine doctor or a naturopath.

Small Intestine Bacterial Overgrowth (SIBO)

Your small intestine shouldn't have all that much bacteria in it, relative to your large intestine. If you end up either with too much in there, or some of the bacteria from your large intestine crawls up into the small intestine, you end up with SIBO (Small Intestine Bacterial Overgrowth).

The bacteria that cause SIBO aren't technically "bad"… there's just too many of them, or they're in the wrong place. Part of the reason this causes a problem is because bacteria's job (in part) is to help us break down the waste left over from our food after we extract all the good stuff. But we extract most of that good stuff in the first part of the small intestine. If the bacteria that shouldn't get to the food particles until much later show up early to the party, they get first dibs… which can mean 1) nutrient deficiencies, and 2) lots of gas and bloating very quickly after eating (either after eating almost anything, or most notably after eating fermentable carbohydrates).

Causes of SIBO:

Unfortunately we don't know for sure what causes SIBO. But there are a few theories:

- **Decreased gut motility.** The slower food moves through your gut, the more easily bacteria in the colon will be able to crawl upstream, as it were. At least that's one theory. I will certainly say patients who have gastroparesis often also have SIBO, and sometimes even higher blood sugar (the precondition for gastroparesis) can do it. I also see this in patients who have had bowel surgeries.
- **Hypothyroidism** will also slow down bowel transit, and that can be a predisposing factor for SIBO (see Chapter 6).
- **Wiping out the good guys.** Your microbiome is the immune system of your gut, and it is your first line of defense against both pathogenic and opportunistic bacteria that can cause you problems.

Lots of antibiotics will lead to flora imbalance (dysbiosis). Proton Pump Inhibitors (PPIs) are actually also antifungals, and these can do it too.

- **Stress.** I know, I know—stress causes everything. And it's true: whatever your weak link is, is likely to snap when you're under a lot of stress. But specifically, stress means you're in "fight-or-flight" mode, and that means less blood flow to your gut (i.e. decreased release of pancreatic enzymes and HCl and bile to help you break down your food, and decreased gut motility) while it instead sends blood to your limbs to help you fight or flee from the perceived danger. So, stress can led to decreased gut motility, which can mean bacteria might have more of an opportunity to crawl upstream.

Signs and Symptoms of SIBO:
- Do you often feel gassy after meals?
- Do you have constipation, diarrhea, or alternation of both?
- Do you feel full after just eating a few bites of food?
- Do probiotics containing inulin or FOS make you gassy?
- Does fiber actually make your constipation worse? (Caveat to this: psyllium has an opposite effect of increasing constipation on about 30% of the population. But if fiber in general has a constipating effect on you, this could be an indication of SIBO.)
- Do your symptoms tend to improve when you take antibiotics?
- Do you have a hard time getting your iron levels up, but haven't ever found a reason for it? (The bacteria themselves can consume some of the iron, accounting for this.)
- Have you had a hard time digesting fats? (These can interfere with bile, which is necessary for the absorption of fat.)
- Do you have acid reflux? (HCl serves as an antibiotic in the stomach, and if it is low, as it often is in acid reflux, this can be one of the causes of SIBO. For this reason, prolonged PPI use can set you up for this too.)
- Do you have excessive belching?
- Do you have increased intestinal permeability (i.e. lots of food allergies?)

Case Study:

Vivien, 36, came to me with bloating and constipation almost all the time, with nearly everything she ate. She felt full after eating a very small amount of food, and she also felt like food "just sat there," particularly heavy protein. Carbs seemed to make the bloating even worse, and too much fat gave her nausea and diarrhea.

We did a SIBO breath test, and found that she had both the methane and the hydrogen producing bacterial overgrowth in her small intestine. Having been in a Facebook support group for those with digestive problems, Vivien knew that Rifaximin, the antibiotic treatment for SIBO, rarely worked the first time, and it was extremely expensive. She opted for an herbal treatment approach, and in her case we chose a highly concentrated garlic extract, since she was not sensitive to FODMAPs (more on this later). We also started her on the Specific Carbohydrate Diet with emphasis on frequent small meals, in order to allow the inflammation in her gut to calm down, and put her on a short-term course of digestive enzymes each time she ate. When she intended to consume high protein, she took HCl, and when she ate a lot of fat, we gave her OxBile as well. I explained that this should not be necessary long-term: once we eliminated the SIBO and interrupted the cycle of inflammation, she ought to be able to eat without the enzymes, HCl, and OxBile. But I told her to continue that part of the protocol for at least 6 weeks.

Meanwhile, lab tests showed that Vivien suffered from subclinical hypothyroidism, which likely served as the precondition that set her up for SIBO in the first place. We put her on NatureThroid, a natural thyroid replacement, and re-checked her thyroid in another 6 weeks.

After the first round of the garlic extract, Vivien felt much better, though not 100%. When she finished it, we put her on Low Dose Erythromycin to encourage gut motility. She stuck with the diet and the digestive support until her thyroid balanced out, but she was amazed at how much better her bowels felt once her thyroid was adequately supported.

She's still careful to eat frequent small meals, but Vivien is now able to cheat on the SCD diet a few times per week without suffering much of a setback. She also no longer needs the digestive aids.

Testing for SIBO:

The small intestine is really hard to reach; endoscopies only reach the upper portion of the small intestine and colonoscopies only reach the bottom portion, leaving a good seventeen feet of it that we can't see without surgery. For that reason, the best way to test for SIBO is with a breath test.

The bacteria that cause SIBO release hydrogen—and in some cases, the hydrogen released can feed a prokaryotic organism called archaea, which then releases methane. So in order to determine whether these organisms are present, you ingest a form of sugar (lactulose is my preference, since humans can't digest it—only bacteria can. But some practitioners use glucose testing instead). Then you breathe into a test tube every twenty minutes for three hours. The levels of hydrogen and/or methane produced will determine the diagnosis.

Treatment for SIBO:

The pharmaceutical treatment for SIBO is a bacteriostatic antibiotic called Rifaximin if only hydrogen is high, and Rifaximin and Neomycin both if methane is also high.

The up side of Rifaximin is that it is not systemically absorbed, but stays within the GI tract. This minimizes its side effect profile. The bacteria are also in the bacteriostatic rather than the bactericidal category, which means they block the reproduction of the bacteria they target, but don't actually wipe them out. This means less gut flora disturbance, if any—in fact, Rifaximin's side effect profile is similar to placebo. Neomycin, another antibiotic recommended for some cases of SIBO in which methane-producing bacteria are also present, also remains local to the gut. I never prescribe Neomycin by itself, however—it's Rifaximin, or Rifaximin plus Neomycin, depending on the type of SIBO.

Unfortunately, there are two main problems with Rifaximin: first, infections tend to recur, and second, it's still under patent and therefore very expensive. Insurance companies have a tendency to deny coverage, and many of my patients have to pay out of pocket. (I usually recommend a discount card to make it more affordable, but even then, at the time of this writing it's still a few hundred dollars for a ten-day course.)

The Herbal Approach

While I probably have more experience treating SIBO with antibiotics, more and more patients either cannot or choose not to go that route. In my experience, the herbs, such as garlic extracts (for those not sensitive to FODMAPs, see below), as well as combinations of berberine and essential oils can also be just as effective as Rifaximin. In one study[12], the specific herbal combination Candibactin AR and BR, and the herbal combinations FC Cidal and Dysbiocide were found to be a bit *more* effective than Rifaximin.

Recurrence of SIBO

Regardless of the treatment approach, SIBO tends to recur. This is usually because the underlying cause of slower bowel motility has not been fully corrected.

Because of the high rate of recurrence, in addition to searching for and treating root causes, I nearly always prescribe some form of prokinetic (an agent that enhances GI motility) after SIBO treatment. Prokinetics help the gut move the way it's supposed to. These can include herbs or prescriptions such as low dose erythromycin (LDE)—technically in the antibiotic category, but at low enough doses it acts as a prokinetic only and lacks antibiotic properties.

It is also necessary to maintain a fairly strict diet that is low in fermentable carbohydrates during treatment. For this I prefer the Specific Carbohydrate Diet, but I do have some patients who have SIBO and do better on the FODMAPs diet instead (see below). In still others, we combine the two.

Have I seen people get completely better? Absolutely. But I will also say that most of those SIBO success cases have also been those where the underlying cause has been identified and corrected.

Avoiding FODMAPS

Sometimes people have reactions to foods that they are not allergic to—rather, they are actually caused by foods in the FODMAPs category. The

FODMAPs acronym stands for Fermentable Oliogosaccharides Disaccharides Monosaccharides And Polyols—all of which are carbohydrates. Fermentable carbs are those that bacteria digest for you.

The FODMAPs diet was developed to deal with functional gastrointestinal symptoms such as bloating, diarrhea, constipation, abdominal pain or discomfort. Here's what those big words in the acronym mean:

- **Oligosaccharides** are fructans (aka prebiotics: the food for the bacteria in your intestines, including FOS and inulin) and galactans (the components of beans and cruciferous veggies that make them hard to digest). These actually make everybody gassy at high enough doses.
- **Disaccharides**: primarily the FODMAP disaccharide is lactose (dairy).
- **Monosaccharides**: the only one that is a FODMAP is fructose (the fruit sugar).
- **Polyols**: these are sugar alcohols, or any sweetener ending in -ol (sorbitol, erythritol, maltitol, etc.) Some of these are naturally occurring in fruit, but they're often used as sweeteners. These, too, will make everyone gassy at a certain threshold.

In case you're wondering what FODMAPS are in English, some of the biggies are dairy, sweeteners, and grains. Certain fruits (peaches, cherries, mangos, melons, avocados, apricots, plums, apples, pears, and nectarines, as well as dried prunes, raisins, currents) and vegetables (asparagus, beets, broccoli, mushrooms, sweet corn, cabbages, peas, onions, garlic, and leeks) can be problematic as well.

If you don't have a super robust gut (if you don't have enough digestive enzymes, for instance, due to leaky gut, or SIBO, or IBD—Crohn's or Ulcerative Colitis), then simpler carbs that ought to get broken down by your digestive system, don't.

When this happens, instead of getting absorbed and used for energy, these carbs hang out in your intestines, and the bacteria that live there (good or bad) will break them down for you. Byproducts of this process include gas and lactic acid—and on top of that, the gas itself can slow down your gut motility (meaning waste moves through you slower than it should).

The shorter the carbohydrate chain, the faster this fermentation process can happen.

Short chain carbs will also draw more water into your intestines, leading to distention and exacerbating the digestive disturbances.

Remember that the oligosaccharides and polyols will cause digestive problems in everyone at a certain threshold—the only question is where that threshold is for you.

Not everyone has a problem with fructose or lactose, though. In order to determine whether you're one who does, you might consider taking a breath test. Like with SIBO, this test can help you find out whether you have difficulty absorbing fructose or lactose. If you don't, then you can consume those foods without an issue.

In many cases, digestive disturbances are relatively simple cases of food allergies, dysbiosis, or candidiasis. These don't generally require long-term fancy diets. Treat the cause, and the problems resolve.

If you have persistent symptoms even after these possibilities have been explored, or if you have SIBO or IBD (Irritable Bowel Disease, such as Crohn's or Ulcerative Colitis), though, you're much more likely to have issues with FODMAPs foods. Like the Specific Carbohydrate Diet (see below), the FODMAPs diet recommends removal of all offending foods for 6-8 weeks, and then beginning a reintroduction challenge with one food at a time once symptoms are gone. This is because even FODMAPs sensitive patients may not have a problem with every single food on the FODMAPs list.

There's a lot of overlap between the Specific Carbohydrate Diet, the GAPS diet (GAPS stands for Gut and Psychology Syndrome, most appropriate for behavioral issues leading back to the gut), and the FODMAPs diet—all of them restrict carbs and minimize beans. But some foods are allowed on one diet plan and disallowed on another. Every body is different, so it may require some testing (breath testing, or removal and reintroduction) to determine the best protocol for you.

Once the underlying inflammation causing the FODMAPs sensitivity is gone, you should be able to go back to eating foods on the FODMAPs list without a problem (as long as you don't way overdo the sugar alcohols and the beans!)

Case Study:

Hank, a very cheerful 70-year-old, came to me with gas, bloating, alternating constipation and diarrhea: all the hallmarks of IBS. Specifically, he felt worse when eating quite a few of the foods on the FODMAPs list (though he didn't call it that), as well as sugar and bread. He told me he had been to the gastroenterologists and the allergists, and nobody could figure out what was wrong with him. He managed his symptoms with stool softeners and Gas-X.

Since Hank's New Patient Paperwork showed that he also suffered from frequent sinus headaches and reflux, I told him that I suspected he had food allergies, and perhaps Leaky Gut Syndrome. I suspected that the inflammation had set him up for dysbiosis, and that when the inflammation is severe enough, it can lead to FODMAPs sensitivities. FODMAPs sensitivities are secondary to the gut inflammation, though: once you heal up the cause of the inflammation, those sensitivities should go away.

We did food allergy testing and a stool culture to identify any dysbiotic organisms. I also put him on a probiotic, and told him to avoid foods in the FODMAPs group until we got the results back. I was surprised when, three weeks later, Hank told me he had been avoiding FODMAPs almost completely! (Very few patients are so compliant.) He said he already felt about 50% better just from these two things.

Hank's test results showed both food allergies and Leaky Gut Syndrome. For the following six weeks, Hank was to avoid foods that triggered his greatest allergic responses, and we put him on glutamine to help repair his intestinal lining. The stool culture showed that he was low in beneficial gut flora, so we put him on even more powerful probiotics than the ones he'd been on after the first visit. He also had overgrowth of an opportunistic yeast, though not candida. We put him on a protocol to avoid sugar and white carbs in addition to the food allergy elimination, too, and on some natural antifungals.

"So, what *can* I eat?" he protested, laughing. I was encouraged to notice that Hank laughed when asking this question. It was clear to me that he was determined to get healthy again.

"Let go of the FODMAPs elimination at this point, and just focus on avoiding the allergens and the foods that feed the yeast for the next six weeks," I advised him. "But stick with the digestive enzymes, too. After six weeks, hopefully you won't need them anymore."

Six weeks later, Hank told me that, to his amazement, his bowels were normal. Not only that, but the post-nasal drip he hadn't even told me about had vanished too. I told him that he could stop the antifungals, drop down to the less aggressive probiotics, and reintroduce the foods we'd eliminated in a rotation fashion.

"After all your hard work, you will likely be able to eat eggs every three days without causing a negative reaction," I told him. "But don't eat them every day. And if you notice symptoms returning with the occasional egg, then listen to your body and stop."

The Specific Carbohydrate Diet

As previously mentioned, there are a number of similarities between the FODMAPs diet and the Specific Carbohydrate Diet (SCD). Because the SCD has a narrower food allowance, it is often used for treating special case types of digestive disturbances. Irritable Bowel Disease is a special case, and needs to be treated as such. While IBS (Irritable Bowel Syndrome) refers just to a collection of symptoms, including bloating and alternating constipation and diarrhea, IBD includes autoimmune conditions Crohn's and Ulcerative Colitis (UC). Both of these are characterized by GI inflammation, and blood and/or mucus in the stool.

The causes of Crohn's and UC are not completely understood, which is essentially the case with all autoimmune conditions. But once the process starts, according to Elaine Gottschall, author of "Breaking the Vicious Cycle,"[6] the cycle goes something like this:

Think of carbs as sugar (which essentially they are—your body converts them into sugar). Your body can absorb simple (single) sugars directly, but complex sugars have to be broken into simple sugars by enzymes, which are found on your intestinal lining, before absorption becomes possible. Then the simple sugars can be absorbed.

If complex carbs don't get broken down (for whatever reason), then they don't get absorbed, and they travel on down through your intestines. Then they come in contact with the bacteria in your gut. These bacteria break down the carbs for you, but they produce two major byproducts: gas (so you feel distended) and acid (which causes inflammation in your intestines). Your body responds to the inflammation by producing mucus to protect itself.

The problem is, the mucus blocks the enzymes in your intestines from coming in contact with other complex carbs you eat. So more complex carbs get turned into gas and acid, producing even more mucus.

In a nutshell: inflammation (from autoimmunity or anything else) → mucus → inability to break down complex carbs → gas and acid → more inflammation → more mucus… and round and round we go.

Gottschall's answer to breaking the cycle (and my clinical experience) is this: you have to interfere with the cycle at the only place where you have some control. And the only part you are directly in control of is what you eat.

If you stop eating carbs that require disaccharide digestive enzymes (mostly grains and processed or canned carbs—that is, carbohydrates that come in a can), the nasty bacteria in your gut have nothing to eat. So instead of producing gas and acid, they starve and die. Gas and intestinal inflammation decrease; therefore mucus production decreases.

The rest of the gut-healing protocol is very similar to the approach for food allergies, and there are almost always a bunch of food allergies secondary to IBD-associated inflammation. These will also need to be addressed. Eventually you should be able to add disaccharides back into your diet, as long as you don't overdo it and continue to avoid foods you're allergic to (which may exacerbate or perpetuate the inflammation as well).

As a side note, some (not all) of these patients also tend towards depression or anxiety. My theory is that, because some 80% of the serotonin in the body is produced in the gut, inflammatory gut conditions can sometimes trigger mental/emotional imbalances. If this is the sole or primary source of the problem, your mood may also improve as the gut heals.

The Autoimmune Protocol (AIP) Diet

Autoimmunity is caused by a confused immune system, and it nearly always goes back to the gut. (Remember that 80% of your immune system lives in the gut!) So it makes perfect sense to address it at the level of the gut. In cases of autoimmunity, some otherwise healthful foods can perpetuate gut inflammation—so I recommend restricting these foods for at least the 6 weeks or so that it generally takes in order to heal up the gut lining.

The Autoimmune Protocol is essentially paleo, which means no grains, no legumes (beans, lentils, etc), no dairy, and nothing refined (sugars, processed veggie oils, or food chemicals).

In addition to this list, the AIP restricts eggs, nuts, seeds, veggies in the nightshade family (potatoes, tomatoes, eggplants, and peppers), and any food with gluten cross-reactivity potential.

What you should eat instead on this diet: grass fed meats and organ meats, lots of seafood (wild caught or otherwise), as many veggies as you can cram in (with the exception of nightshades), fermented foods, and bone broth.

The AIP Diet is a grain free diet. I certainly have some patients whose guts are so inflamed that they cannot tolerate grains at all, nor starchy veggies like potatoes. These tend to be SIBO patients or patients with Irritable Bowel Disease, such as Crohn's or Ulcerative Colitis, for the most part, and this is one reason why they do best on the Specific Carbohydrate Diet. The reason for this goes back to the "vicious cycle" of inflammation, as described by Elaine Gottschall (see the Specific Carbohydrate Diet explanation, above). Grains, even whole grains, are relatively simple carbs and can set off the inflammatory process. If the gut is inflamed, as it always is in the case of autoimmunity, grains will exacerbate this process. So avoidance is best, at least until healing can occur.

Legumes are also restricted in the AIP diet. Legumes are a great source of protein, and generally very nutrient-dense. The biggest problem with them that I can see is that 1) they contain phytic acid (an anti-nutrient of sorts: it binds other nutrients and prevents you from absorbing them; you can get around this by soaking your beans first though), 2) they tend to shift the immune system into Th1 dominance (meaning they can exacerbate organ-specific autoimmunity), and 3) they're one of the FODMAPs, which means they are very likely to cause problems for people whose guts are inflamed. That said, as mentioned previously, I've yet to meet a patient who is sensitive to everything on the FODMAPs list. It's always a trial-and-error process (though I will say beans are a BIG one that tend to make most people gassy).

I do see a decent number of patients who also turn out to be sensitive to legumes on food allergy testing—so eliminating legumes on this protocol follows the same logic as an allergy elimination diet.

Dairy is also restricted on the AIP diet, and it, too, has a high allergenic potential. It also tends to encourage Th1 dominance, potentially exacerbating organ-specific autoimmunity.

Additionally, dairy can cross-react with gluten, another very common sensitivity. That means if you're sensitive to gluten (i.e. your body is creating antibodies against it), you may end up reacting to dairy also just because there are certain segments of the dairy antigen that look very much like the gluten antigen. So even if you're not creating antibodies against dairy itself, your body might still react as if it were.

By the way, if you're gluten sensitive, this might also be the case with oats, millet, soy, corn, rice, yeast, and potatoes. But since those are mostly grains, legumes, or nightshades anyway, it doesn't eliminate anything new.

Overall, I think the diet is an excellent way to cover your bases and make sure you're not eating anything that has the potential to exacerbate gut inflammation on a number of different fronts. The foods that are recommended on this diet are very nutrient-dense, as well. For someone with autoimmunity, and especially someone who has not undergone food allergy testing to determine which foods actually do cause him or her problems, it's a good option. My only concern is that, for patients who might say, "But what *can* I eat?," it might be unnecessarily restrictive. I disagree that everyone (even everyone with autoimmunity) necessarily needs to avoid nuts, seeds, nightshades, or eggs. If you haven't had testing to determine whether you're one of the people who does or not, then as with a traditional allergy elimination diet, it's safest to just cut them out while you're trying to heal, and reintroduce them later while monitoring your body for a return of symptoms.

I would not recommend this protocol for someone with yeast overgrowth or SIBO, only because of the recommendation to consume large amounts of fermented foods (which can tend to exacerbate bacterial or yeast overgrowth), and the lack of restriction on fruit (ditto), while foods that should not cause any issues for these people are restricted.

Gut inflammation of all kinds can lead to food allergies, certainly. But they can also lead to histamine intolerance. This is another kind of inflammation that looks very much like food allergies, yet with a very different mechanism of action.

Histamine

Histamine intolerance occurs due to increased levels of histamine, secondary to poorly functioning or overwhelmed enzymes that can't break it down fast enough. In order to understand this, let's first consider how histamine is supposed to work, and then how the overwhelm can occur.

Histamine is an amino acid with several important functions in the body. The one we are familiar with is its role in the immune system: histamine gets released in response to an infection or injury to help attract white blood cells to clean up the problem. Dysfunction of this process results in allergies: inappropriate immune response to an otherwise harmless "friend" (like foods, pets, pollen, etc) rather than a foe (a bacteria, virus, fungus, or external injury).

Histamine also functions as a neurotransmitter—specifically, it helps stimulate wakefulness, which is the reason why many of us notice that taking a Benadryl (an H1 histamine blocker) can make us drowsy.

In the stomach, histamine is also required for the first step in the release of gastric acid (HCl). This is why some of the most popular classes of drugs to block stomach acid are H2 (histamine receptor) blockers. (Ironically, as mentioned in Chapter 1, most of the time GERD or reflux is due to stomach acid that is too low, not too high, and very often this goes back to food allergies. The meds do help with symptom suppression though.)

Two different enzymes are responsible for breaking histamine down, depending on where it is in the body: histamine N-methyltransferase (HMT) in the Central Nervous System as well as in other tissues, and Diamine Oxidase (DAO) primarily in the gut, as well as in other tissues.

Histamine in Your Food

Some foods naturally contain histamine, and some facilitate the release of histamine. Here are the big ones:

- **Veggies:** spinach, avocados, tomatoes, and white potatoes
- **Fruits**: citrus, strawberries, cherries, bananas, pineapple, kiwi, papaya, mango, raspberries, pears.
- **Animal protein**: anything processed (bacon, sausage, salami, pepperoni, etc); shellfish; fish that is not freshly caught. (If it's frozen it's probably fine. If it's been sitting in your fridge for a few days, it likely will release histamine.)
- **Fermented foods**: including yogurt, vinegar, alcohol, mushrooms
- **Nuts and seeds**: all of them
- **Sugar**
- **Chocolate**
- **Cheese**
- **Yeast**

All of these foods require the DAO enzyme in order to get broken down. In a healthy intestinal tract, that is no problem; but in the presence of gut inflammation, it can mean trouble.

Histamine Intolerance (or too much histamine)

DAO (diamine oxidase) levels can be used as a marker for decreased intestinal integrity[1]. Lower DAO means increased circulating histamine levels… and increased circulating histamine levels throughout the body can mean any of the following symptoms:

- Insomnia
- Arrhythmia or unusual heartbeats
- Rashes and hives
- Headaches and migraines
- Vertigo
- Flushing
- Nasal congestion
- Swelling
- Abdominal cramping

Generally histamine intolerance is secondary to gut inflammation, which can be due to leaky gut syndrome, SIBO, Irritable Bowel Disease, Irritable Bowel Syndrome, gluten intolerance or Celiac Disease.

Some medications can also lower DAO function, particularly those that hit the gut. These include ibuprofen and aspirin, many antidepressants, and (ironically) both H1 and H2 blockers.

Treating Histamine Intolerance
In most cases, a low histamine diet, or eating high histamine foods with a DAO supplement, will lower the overall histamine levels enough for symptoms to subside.

But the real treatment is to address the reason why histamine levels increased in the first place. This root cause usually goes back to the gut.

Okay, so let's assume you're done with the appropriate specialty diet for you: allergy avoidance, Specific Carbohydrate, FODMAPs, Autoimmune Protocol, Candida Protocol, etc—and you're ready to transition to a basic "healthy" diet. Whether you decide to go vegan or vegetarian or paleo or ketogenic or just try to eat whole foods, there is one major food category (if it can be called a category) that you will especially need to watch out for.

The Worst Food for Dysbiosis (and Western Disease in General)
According to Weston Price, a dentist who researched traditional diets around the world in the 1930s, the culprits for Western diseases are white flour, sugar, and

processed vegetable fats.[3] Traditional diets ranging from almost entirely plant based to almost entirely animal based *all* produced healthy populations; it was not until the Western processed foods infiltrated those societies that their health began to decline.

Many people think of 'sugar' as the white granules that we stir in our coffee or add to our cookie recipe. Although that *is* sugar, doctors and scientists have a much broader definition, using something called the glycemic index. This is a measure of how quickly a particular food turns to sugar in the body. Which of the following do you believe delivers the highest calorie-for-calorie sugar hit (glycemic index) in the body?

1) Donut
2) Ice cream
3) Baked white potato
4) Jelly beans

If you guessed #3, you are correct. The glycemic index for the donut is 76, for ice cream it is 60, and for jelly beans it is 80. The white potato has a glycemic index (sugar hitting the bloodstream) of 85!

The benchmark for these numbers is pure glucose, assigned a glycemic index of 100. Everything else is assigned a number relative to that. As you can tell, at the top of the glycemic index list are all things white, especially processed white flour (including white bread, pancakes, and pastries), most processed white grains (including white rice, instant oatmeal, popcorn, and most cereals), and white potatoes, especially potato products (including french fries, potato chips, and instant mashed potatoes).

Think of sugar as quick energy. It can get converted into the currency your body uses for energy very quickly. But your blood can only accommodate a few tablespoons of sugar at a time. So your body tries to get rid of excess sugar from the bloodstream in order to minimize this process. Sugar has to get inside the cells in order to get out of the blood. Sugar can't just rush into the cells though—it has to have the key to get in. The key is insulin, and it gets produced from the pancreas in response to high sugar in the bloodstream. This works great for a while… but problems come in when this cycle is repeated too often, too long. Like a drug addict needing a bigger dose to achieve the same high, the body will start to require more and more insulin to keep up with your sugar intake. Eventually, the pancreas can't keep up with the demand. (This leads to Insulin Resistance and Diabetes.) Once the sugar gets inside the cells, it can't be stored in its present form—it has to be converted from "quick" energy into "potential" energy—fat (or more precisely, triglycerides.) So sugar also leads to obesity. Other prevalent Western diseases linked to sugar consumption include cancer (and cancer cells consume sugar as energy before the rest of the body, so eating sugar will feed cancer cells), dementia and Alzheimer's disease, IBS of course (sugar feeds several of the dysbiotic flora contributing to gas, bloating, and constipation), and many more.[4]

Even knowing all this, many people find it hard to stop eating sugar. This is because sugar is an addiction—just like alcohol, smoking, and drugs. A research study found that sugar produces a chemical in the brain called enkephalins, which work much like opiates (including heroin, morphine, and oxycontin)—that is, they stimulate the release of dopamine.[11] Most other addictions do the same thing: dopamine is the neurotransmitter in the brain linked to pleasure and reward.

Are you addicted to sugar? Here are a few questions to ask yourself in order to find out: Do you use sugar and foods that act like sugar (with a high glycemic index) to make you feel better after a bad day? Do you crave sugar or high glycemic index foods? Do you think lower glycemic index foods taste bland, and feel the need to add sweetener? Have you ever tried to avoid sugar and found that either you couldn't, or once you tasted something sweet you felt compelled to consume all of it? Do you use sugar, and foods that act like sugar, as a reward for yourself? If you answered yes to several of those questions, you are far from alone! Although it is not an easy habit to break (they never are), it is one of the very best choices that you can make for your health.

One tip for the emotional eaters out there: if you find that you crave the comfort that sweet foods bring, you are probably self-medicating for the serotonin boost they provide. If this is the case, consider trying L-Tryptophan or 5-HTP, the precursors for serotonin. You can take about 50 mg of 5-HTP or 1000 mg of L-Tryptophan (one or the other, not both) in the afternoon or the evening, on an empty stomach, and see if this helps to offset the cravings. If instead you crave the sense of reward or fulfillment that comes from sweet foods, you might do better with a precursor to dopamine, like DL-Phenylalanine or L-Tyrosine. You can take one of these (about 1000 mg) on an empty stomach in the morning or early afternoon (not at night, since they can keep you awake).

If you are on any antidepressant or psychotropic medications, or if you suffer from bipolar disorder, please talk to your health care practitioner before starting these, as they can affect your neurotransmitter balance.

Sodas: A Particularly Bad Sugar Source

On the topic of sugar… many people that have an addiction to sodas, which can certainly set you up for dysbiosis. Sodas can be an exceptionally difficult habit to kick, because they are everywhere.

Regular sodas can have up to 50-80 grams of sugar per can. (Context: a regular size Snickers bar has 30 grams!) While adults get about 7% of their calories from soda, teenagers get some 13% from soda.

High Fructose Corn Syrup, one of the most common sweeteners in sodas, is especially nasty. While the body gets to choose whether it wants to use glucose (regular sugar) for energy or store it for future use (as fat), fructose bypasses this regulatory step and goes straight to fat (more on this below). This means that it increases BMI and triglycerides, but doesn't curb your appetite at all. It's also six times as sweet as regular sugar—so in a sense, it "spoils" your taste for good, natural food.

Soda also has a possible relationship to ADHD symptoms: a huge influx of sugar requires a huge output of insulin, which then leads to an equally fast sugar crash. The resulting hypoglycemia (low blood sugar) symptoms include shakiness, irritability, low energy and attention span, and sugar craving (so it perpetuates the cycle of poor food choices). And of course, the point of this chapter: sugar is also the primary food for intestinal yeast. If you eat a lot of sugar over a long enough period of time, and/or if you also have a poor gut flora balance to begin with, you may end up with candida overgrowth or overgrowth of other dysbiotic flora. You could end up with bloating, alternating constipation and diarrhea, as well as brain fog and poor memory and concentration.

Remember that you cannot save yourself from the dangers of soda by switching to a diet variety, which instead includes artificial sweeteners such as Splenda (sucralose), Equal or NutraSweet (aspartame), and Sweet 'N Low (saccharin). Collectively these chemicals are associated with leukemia, brain tumors, breast cancer, bladder cancer, uterine and ovarian cancer, skin cancer, immune dysfunction, DNA damage, preterm delivery, and neurological problems. (Personally I'd rather be overweight and inattentive!) However, people who drink diet sodas are statistically even heavier than those who drink regular sodas. At first, this appears to make no sense—glucose (sugar) can get directly converted into triglycerides which get stored as fat, but artificial sweeteners cannot. But as mentioned in Chapter 1, artificial sweeteners disrupt your gut flora, which leads to weight gain as well as dysbiosis.

Beyond the pick-your-poison sweeteners, sodas are full of artificial colors (you now know these cause cancer and hyperactivity) and artificial flavors.[12] They also have toxic preservatives and sometimes, from a chemical reaction, benzene. In addition, because of their phosphoric acid content, they lead to mineral loss.[13] Then there's the caffeine, which in excess can cause its own set of problems.

So instead of soda, instead choose water, unsweetened tea (or sweetened with stevia, a little bit of honey, or even real cane sugar as long as you don't go to town with it), small amounts of coffee (a cup or at most two won't hurt most of you), diluted fruit juice (to cut the sugar concentration), coconut water, or carbonated flavored water.

Is Fructose a Healthy Sugar?

Fructose is the sugar found in fruit. "If it's in fruit, it must be healthy, right?" many people wonder. As a general rule, nothing that God made is unhealthy across the board. There are certain circumstances under which eating too much fruit might be a bad idea (for instance, a patient with intestinal candidiasis, or insulin resistance), though. In those cases, limiting fruit to 1-2 pieces per day and going with the ones lower in sugar is wise until the condition is reversed.

But when fructose is extracted from fruit and used as a sweetener for other things, it is definitely not healthy, because it is not properly regulated by the body.

When you ingest glucose (or a carb that can be broken down into glucose), it enters a ten-step biochemical process called glycolysis as one of three cycles to convert the glucose into your body's energy currency, called ATP. At step 5 of glycolysis, your body gets to decide, based on its current needs, whether the glucose should be sent to storage (where it'll end up as body fat) or whether it should be used as energy.

Fructose, however, enters glycolysis just after this regulatory step. Instead of continuing through glycolysis for energy production, it goes straight to storage (fat).

Because it bypasses the regulatory step, your body never asks itself the question, "Do I need energy right now or am I full?"

Leptin is a hormone secreted by adipose tissue (fat cells) that tells you you're full. (Its opposite hormone is called ghrelin, which tells you you're hungry. You can remember this because the word ghrelin sounds like a stomach growling.) When your body detects that you have plenty of glucose (via insulin, see below) and your energy capacity is high (ie. you have adequate ATP), leptin will send the signal, "Stop eating, we have enough right now!"

But fructose doesn't trigger insulin, and therefore it doesn't trigger leptin. So you keep eating, gaining the extra as fat.

Because fructose doesn't trigger insulin, you'd think this would make it less likely to cause insulin resistance than too much glucose might do. However, high fructose consumption is strongly associated with development of insulin resistance in animals[14], and the data suggests the same process occurs in humans. This may be because fructose turns into fat in the liver more readily than does glucose, and NAFLD (Non-Alcoholic Fatty Liver Disease) is strongly correlated with insulin resistance. It may be because fructose consumption leads to central obesity (since it goes straight to storage), and central obesity leads to insulin resistance. The process isn't fully understood, but the connections are certainly there.

Let me clarify: *in a piece of fruit, fructose is not bad for you.* There's not that much of it, relative to the fiber and all the nutrients you're getting in the fruit. (If you eat nothing *but* fruit, though, you can potentially set yourself up for candidiasis or nutrient deficiencies.)

Fruit juice (or fruit concentrate), however, is the fruit with none of the fiber, which slows the release of the fructose into your bloodstream— so it's a whopping dose of sugar all rushing into storage at once. Likewise, products "sweetened with fruit juice" may sound natural, but they are not healthy. They're not as bad as, say, aspartame, but you're not doing yourself any favors.

The bottom line is that you should skip anything sweetened with fruit juice… or at least consume it as sparingly as you would regular sugar. Minimize fruit juices as beverages, or dilute them with water. (And if you are wondering about agave, as natural as it sounds, it is 90% fructose. You're better off choosing honey.)

There are other things that can cause dysbiosis besides your food choices, of course. Quite a few different popular classes of medications can do it, too.

Contraceptive Side Effects

Birth control medications are a very popular type of prescription drug. Many doctors will prescribe hormone-based birth control pills in an effort to regulate your cycle. These are often effective, and while many women do fine on them, they do have a tendency to disrupt gut flora. In fact, I have had a few patients with dysbiosis that refused to clear as long as they continued on birth control. For the purposes of this chapter, that alone is something to keep in mind.

There are other long-term consequences too, though, such as increased risk of certain cancers and of stroke (especially for women over 35 who smoke).

One formerly popular hormonal contraceptive pill is Yasmin. Its side effects have spurred lawsuits. Yasmin's side effects include breast pain or tenderness, headaches, non-menstrual vaginal bleeding, irregular menstrual periods, nausea and/or vomiting, longer and/or heavier menstrual periods, general tiredness or weakness, chills, *candidiasis (yeast infections—which always means there's overgrowth of yeast in the gut too)*, urinary tract infections, upper respiratory infections, difficulty breathing, dizziness, fever, itching, loss of appetite or increased appetite, pain in the chest, groin, or legs, rash, slurred speech, sudden loss of coordination, sudden severe limb weakness, halitosis, vision changes, vomiting of blood, crying, decreased libido, delusions and/or combativeness, false sense of well-being, irritability, depression, emotional overreaction, mood swings, weight gain, acne, hair loss, hypertension, increased serum potassium levels, jaundice, amenorrhea, melasma, edema, exacerbations of Lupus, porphyria, and chorea, diminished lactation, flu syndrome, tooth disorder, infection, aggravation of varicose veins, heart attack, stroke, vascular thrombosis (blood clots) or embolism, changes in plasma lipid profiles and carbohydrate metabolism, lowered glucose tolerance levels, gallbladder disease, esophageal ulceration, retinal thrombosis, optic neuritis, osteonecrosis (bone death), and benign migratory glossitis. There are also, as mentioned previously, associations with breast cancer, cervical cancer, and liver cancer.[15]

My $0.02: if you are considering birth control options, look into Natural Family Planning, as described in Toni Weschler's excellent book, *Taking Charge of Your Fertility*. Birth control technically is not "natural," but this is the closest thing I've found. It requires you to learn your cycles and work with your body rather than against it, to either achieve or avoid pregnancy.

Side Effects of Antacid Treatment

Antacids directly disrupt the digestion process, so it's no wonder that they can have far-reaching side effects upon the gut, including dysbiosis. For instance, here is a listing of side effects for Dexilant, a drug used for serious reflux: diarrhea, abdominal pain, nausea, respiratory infection, vomiting, flatulence, and, with long term use, vitamin B12 deficiency. The serious reactions are typically a general hypersensitivity reaction or anaphylaxis, Stevens-Johnson syndrome, toxic epidermal necrolysis, interstitial nephritis, bone fractures, diarrhea associated with a C. difficile problem, and, with long term use, hypomagnesemia or atrophic gastritis.

Even if you manage to avoid the more severe side effects, in order to truly correct dysbiosis, it's important to taper off of PPIs or H2 blockers, as they tend to be an obstacle to cure. I always taper, since stopping cold turkey tends to lead to rebound acidity, and in very severe cases in which patients have been medicated for years, we go very slowly indeed. But we don't even start the process until we've corrected the underlying reason for the reflux. Nine times out of ten, this goes back to food allergies (see Chapters 1 and 2), although sometimes it can be a hiatal hernia, low HCl and/or gastritis, in addition to or instead of food allergies.

Case Study:

Heidi came to me after her severe reflux led her to seek a Nissen Fundoplication surgical correction. Sadly, her reflux continued even after the surgery, and she described the pain as sometimes up to 9 or 10 out of 10 in severity. So many foods caused her symptoms to flare that by the time I saw her, she was really only eating about ten foods, all of which were either meat or vegetables. She had been on Dexilant for years, and she was at the highest dose; there was nowhere else for her to go for symptom control.

The process for Heidi was slow. We started with food allergy testing, and since she also had gastritis, we put her on nutrients to help heal up her gut lining: N-Acetyl Glucosamine, slippery elm, deglycyrrhizinated licorice (DGL), zinc carnosine, and aloe vera juice. Given the severity of her symptoms and the length of her treatment, I was almost certain she also had dysbiosis, so we did a stool culture. Sure enough, her good gut flora was almost nonexistent, and she had yeast overgrowth as well as several different types of pathogenic bacteria. We put her on a protocol to try to balance her gut flora, but I knew it would never fully resolve until we got her off of the PPIs, which would be some time.

Her symptoms improved little by little, but what actually made the biggest difference was the addition of a homeopathic remedy that fit both her symptoms and her constitution. Once we did that, at each return visit, her improvement was remarkable. Once reflux pain was down to 1-2/10 more often than not, we started the taper process. In her case, we had to switch her to a different PPI (omeprazole) so that we could taper her off through a compounding pharmacy at minute step-down amounts. Each time she experienced breakthrough reflux, we'd slow down and add in more support. As she could tolerate them, we reintroduced more foods into her diet, continuing to avoid those which showed up on her food allergy panel until she was off of omeprazole entirely. We kept her on very high dose probiotics, knowing that they'd be working at cross purposes until the PPI was completely gone.

Heidi continues to do well—at the time of this writing, she is completely off of omeprazole, her diet has expanded, and reflux symptoms are now quite rare.

Antibiotics and Dysbiosis

Perhaps the only thing harder on digestion than antacids are antibiotics. How big a deal is one round of antibiotics? With some antibiotics, it's enough to disrupt your gut flora for a whole year. For months after taking a full course of ciprofloxacin, clindamycin, amoxicillin or minocycline, participants were found to have decreased bifidobacillus, the organisms that produce butyrate (food for the colon, helping to prevent colon cancer and helpful to heal up any kind of inflammation in the colon, like Crohn's and Ulcerative Colitis). Diversity of gut flora also declined for up to 12 months with ciprofloxacin (not surprising because that's like the nuclear warhead of antibiotics). Amoxicillin (in the penicillin family) didn't affect diversity much, but it did lead to antibiotic resistant genes in the bacteria.[16]

Diversity creates a sort of checks-and-balances system that prevents a single genetic weakness in the gut flora from wreaking havoc and leading you to become far more susceptible to infection. Less diversity means greater susceptibility to illness.

Your gut, we are realizing more and more, is the gateway not just to pathogenic illnesses, but also to noninfectious gut disorders like allergies and autoimmunity. It's also the key to protecting against these ailments.

Microbes adapt to their environments just like we do. Their goal is to survive, just like ours is. It's essentially a war. How long it takes for bacteria to develop resistance to an antibiotic depends on how long and how often that bacteria is exposed to a drug.

At this point, according to the CDC, bacteria are now becoming resistant to the drugs we have faster than we can create new drugs to which they haven't yet adapted.[11] This is partly because of over-prescribing, and partly because we're not coming out with new antibiotics nearly as often as we used to. (Antibiotics, which are prescribed for short courses only, are less profitable for drug companies than drugs people might be expected to stay on long term.)

This is why it's important to save the "big guns" (like ciprofloxacin) for cases that really need it… and to limit the prescription of antibiotics in general only to cases that truly require them.

More often than not, some heavy duty immune support (food, supplements, fasting, sleeping more) is all it takes! In cases where some intervention is required (but not necessarily "The Big Guns"), there are very powerful antimicrobial herbal options.

Dysbiosis and candidiasis require specific protocols for elimination, which have been discussed above. For more help tailoring these to your specific case, I highly recommend finding a functional medicine or naturopathic doctor.

Once you've done that, though, it's a good idea to add in a few extra nutrients to ensure that you can maintain your new and improved gut function.

Dysbiosis and Gut Healing Nutrients

As part of restoring gut health, I recommend that you pay special attention to your cell membranes. Historically the "brain" of the cell was considered to be its nucleus, and cell walls were considered to be the "skin." But if you remove the nucleus from a cell, it can still function just fine—it just can't reproduce (implying that the nucleus is more like the cell's reproductive organ than its brain.) But if you remove the cell's membrane, the cell dies immediately. For this reason (and others) many researchers now refer to the cell membrane as the cell's brain.

Cell membranes are like gates, and the receptors dotted along the membrane are like gatekeepers. They require a certain "password" or key in order to open and let a particular substance inside the cell—not just anybody gets in. But the "gate" has to be fluid enough to allow the gatekeepers to do their jobs properly, and also to let out the internal waste left over from cellular processes. Healthy cell gates will let in nutrients and oxygen, let in cell signals, let in glucose for energy, let in neurotransmitters, maintain proper nerve conduction, and let the "trash" out.

From the standpoint of gut health, healthy cell membranes are critical. Unhealthy membranes also lead to inflammation, and inflammation is exactly what we are trying to get rid of.

Essential fatty acids are one important component for keeping the cell membrane healthy. Fifty percent of your cell membranes are made up of phosphatidylcholine, a phospholipid (fatty acids bound to a backbone of phosphates).

Phosphatidylcholine is found in eggs, milk, soybeans, mustard, peanuts, liver, and sunflowers, but you can also take it as a supplement (and for some people this is necessary, since eggs, milk, soy, and peanuts are all very common allergens). All commercial phosphatidylcholine comes from lecithin, which is usually a byproduct of soybean oil (GMO unless otherwise stated), although it can come from sunflower oil as well. Lecithin does contain phosphatidylcholine, but it contains other phospholipids as well—so percentage-wise, you're not getting as much as if you took a pure version. My preference is a liposomal version of phosphatidylcholine (not choline, not lecithin) derived from sunflowers. It's highly absorbable, it's a much higher percentage of the component you want, and it avoids the GMO issue from soy.

Another valuable gut healing nutrient is **glutamine**. Glutamine is the main "food" for your small intestine. It helps it to knit back together, though it does need to be dosed at about 4-5 grams daily in order to have this effect. Not everyone does well on glutamine: in some, particularly those with severe dysbiosis, it can convert to glutamate (an excitatory neurotransmitter) and cause hyperactivity. But in the vast majority of my leaky gut patients, it is the key to allowing the rest of the treatment to "take." Some of these patients choose to take **bone broth** instead, which contains a high percentage of glutamine. I also occasionally prescribe **IgG immunoglobulins** directly to help heal up the gut lining for some of my very sensitive patients.

And of course, **probiotics**. Find a probiotic with a 50/50 ratio of bifidobacillus to lactobacillus, and at least 20 billion organisms per day. If you have SIBO, it's important to choose a probiotic containing lactobacillus only, until your gut has fully healed.

Gut Healing Nutrient	Purpose	Dosing
Glutamine	food for the small intestine; helps to restore intestinal integrity	4-5 grams daily for the duration of treatment
Phosphatidylcholine	helps to restore the integrity of the gut's cell membranes	700 mg 1-3 times daily for the duration of treatment
Probiotics	restore the good gut microflora to help fight off foreign invaders and help you digest your food	20 billion organisms nightly, 50/50 ratio of bifidobacillus to lactobacillus. This is your ongoing dose; doses up to 450 billion during treatment are sometimes appropriate.
Bone Broth	A rich dietary source of glutamine	1 cup per day for the duration of treatment
CandidaStat	A combination of nutrients and herbs that kills yeast. It's the most effective product I've found for this purpose.	2 caps three times daily for the first bottle, and then drop down to 1 cap three times daily for the rest of the 6 weeks.

Grapefruit Seed Extract	A powerful antimicrobial to which most dysbiotic organisms test sensitive on stool cultures	1 cap three times daily for 2-4 weeks
Allimax	A potent garlic extract with antimicrobial effects. Helpful for most dysbiotic organisms, and SIBO, provided no FODMAP sensivity	1 cap three times daily for 10-20 days
Candibactin AR and Candibactin BR	A combination of herbs and essential oils, shown to be as effective as Rifaximin for treating SIBO	2 tablets of each three times daily for 20 days

The Take-Home Message

Dysbiosis can be yeast overgrowth, it can be bacterial overgrowth, it can be SIBO, or it can be secondary to an underlying problem (such as autoimmunity, Irritable Bowel Disease, food allergies, and leaky gut syndrome.) If it's secondary to an underlying problem, it's important to identify what that problem is and address it either before or while you are dealing with dysbiosis itself.

Healing dysbiosis depends upon the cause.

If it's yeast overgrowth: eliminate sugar and white carbohydrates, add a natural antifungal (such as CandidaStat, or Grapefruit seed extract, or Allimax), and add a probiotic. Be aware that you can end up with die-off while taking antifungals (meaning your immune system attacks all at once and you feel like you're coming down with the flu). If this happens, activated charcoal is a great binder to help you feel better fast. (For this purpose, I'd do activated charcoal at 2 caps three times daily for five days, with 8 oz water each time. The water will keep from constipating you. Also, be aware that activated charcoal will turn your stool black; don't freak out about it.)

If it's SIBO, go on the Specific Carbohydrate Diet, perhaps picking and choosing some of the additional FODMAPs that also trigger you. Go on a lactobacillus-only probiotic, and consider Candibactin-AR and Candibactin-BR. You will very likely also need to see a functional medicine practitioner to help with assessing the underlying cause of your SIBO, and to prescribe an appropriate prokinetic for you to minimize the likelihood of recurrence.

If it's a bacterial organism (or even a parasite), it's valuable to have a comprehensive stool culture, such as those done by Doctor's Data (I like Comprehensive Stool and Parasitology x3) or Genova Diagnostics, which will tell you what the organism is and how to kill it. These will also tell you whether you have imbalanced gut flora, which can help with creating your treatment plan. As mentioned above—if it's a bacterial organism, the vast majority are sensitive to Grapefruit Seed Extract in my experience.

Chapter

5

TOXIC BUILDUP FROM STRESS

hemicals and other toxins are certainly important for gut health, but I would be remiss if I did not discuss the topic of stress. Stress is *the* most pervasive toxin we have. No one is immune from it, and even people who live otherwise "clean" lives can suffer from it. When you're stressed, whatever your weak link is has a tendency to blow (which, if you're reading this book, is most likely your gut). Most of us have experienced abdominal discomfort when anticipating a negative medical report, or getting a grade back on a test; for most of us, the emotion-gut connection is very apparent. Long-term, cortisol imbalance (the stress hormone) can also weaken the gut lining and render you susceptible to inflammation, and this can set you up for leaky gut syndrome, allergies, sensitivity to FODMAPs, dysbiosis, and potentially even autoimmunity.

An estimated 75-90% of all visits to Primary Care Physicians are for stress-related complaints or disorders. Stress has been linked to *all* of the leading causes of death, including heart disease and cancer.

Clearly, proper stress management techniques are absolutely fundamental to your health.

To start, it is essential that you know that stress is not what happens *to* us; it's the way our bodies react to it. Next, you need to identify where the stress is coming from. Some stress is self-inflicted or can be otherwise mitigated. Some you can't do much about, and you just have to survive it. Hopefully this will only last for a season; if it's a long-term problem, it might be time to take a good hard look at your priorities. But if we supply our bodies and our minds with positive, healthful influences, we will be much better equipped to deal with the challenges of life.

The Early Signs of Stress

You may first notice the effects of stress on your mind. The common culture of the American workplace, filled with myriad distractions, high pressure, noise, and multitasking leads us to an environmental product called Attention Deficit Trait (ADT). People working with ADT find it difficult to prioritize, stay organized, and manage time effectively. This leads to a downward spiral of decreasing productivity, and increasing angst. Very commonly patients with apparent ADT tell me that they "can't shut off their brains," especially at night—they lie awake for hours, or wake in the wee hours of the morning, trying to solve the problems that confront them during the day. They tend to be anxious and irritable, and while some take this irritability out on their coworkers or loved ones, others will turn it inward, blaming themselves.

Fortunately, there is a better answer than Ritalin (or Xanax, or Prozac). Think of these symptoms as an early warning system. If the problem is your environment, medicating yourself so that you can better cope with it is sort of like turning off the fire alarm when your house is on fire, instead of grabbing the extinguisher. Eventually the house is still going to burn down, whether you sleep through it or not!

If you choose to ignore the warning symptoms, your stress will continue to grow and will eventually start impacting you physically.

How Stress Affects Your Body

Your adrenals are these two pyramid-shaped glands that sit on top of your kidneys. They've got several jobs, but the biggest is to help your body cope with stress.

If you were to get attacked by a bear, without sparing the critical seconds necessary to talk to your Central Nervous System (CNS), the core of your adrenals flood your body with adrenaline directly—it's an automatic response. This makes your heart race and your bronchioles in your lungs dilate. It provides your muscles with immediate blood flow (oxygen and glucose for energy) to get away quickly or fight, if it comes to that. The adrenaline also overrides this little "gatekeeper" in your muscles called the golgi tendon organ. Its job is to prevent over-strain on the muscles. If you're fighting for your life, over-strain isn't that important—and this is the reason why a flood of adrenaline can allow people to perform superhuman feats.

After you've either killed the bear or escaped, the outside of your adrenals produces another hormone called cortisol. Due to the rush of adrenaline, you've just consumed massive sugar reserves (so now you're probably shaky and hypoglycemic), your blood pressure and heart rate are really high, and your body has totally neglected normal life maintenance stuff like digesting your food and repairing your tissues. Cortisol helps to restore this balance. It encourages the breakdown of glycogen (stored glucose) and gluconeogenesis (production of new glucose from fat in the liver). It redirects blood flow to repair tissues and digest food. It's basically the natural steroid of your body (the equivalent of prednisone, though not nearly as strong), so it's an anti-inflammatory as well... and also an immune suppressant. (This is because you shouldn't spare the energy to fight off a cold when you're busy running from a bear. Survival takes precedence.)

This fight-or-flight system is only designed to be activated in extreme crisis, but a lot of us live in crisis all the time. We're in this constant cycle of "I have to get this done or I'll lose my job!" or "I have to get the kids to school, and then I have to clean the house, and why is everything dirty, and I have to cook, and go to the grocery and..." or "I don't have time for this, get the *$%^& out of my way!" (Don't pretend you don't know what I'm talking about. I know you do.)

The result of this is that our adrenal glands get worn out and we end up with something called Adrenal Fatigue. This is the point at which gut issues can start to occur, among other chronic problems.

Acute (Early Stage) Adrenal Fatigue

The long-term effect of an acutely stressful situation (one that's only started in the last few weeks to few months) is going to be high circulating cortisol, which will suppress your immune function. As anyone who has used topical corticosteroids like hydrocortisone knows, cortisol also thins the skin—and it weakens tissues in general. (This is why cortisone injections may help inflammatory pain in the short-term, but over time they will weaken fascia and exacerbate the original problem.)

What this means: if you're in a stressful period in your life, you'll have more anti-inflammatory cortisol circulating to begin with, which increases the chances of getting sick. Then let's say you *get* sick—that's another stressor, which requires initially more adrenaline, and then more cortisol. Given the amount of your baseline cortisol, you'll have a harder time bouncing back.

Or if you're in that same stressful period and then you have a hard workout, this too will initially spike more adrenaline and then more cortisol... but the higher cortisol "set point" from before the workout will hinder your body's ability to recruit the necessary cytokines to heal the muscle microtears from the workout.

The very same thing applies to surgery: in itself, surgery is a major stressor, and it requires sufficient cortisol to counteract the adrenaline spike. But if you had too much cortisol going into surgery, this will hinder your body's healing process afterwards.

Late Stage Adrenal Fatigue

Later stages of adrenal stress occur when the adrenals are no longer able to produce enough cortisol to compensate for the adrenaline surges. This stage is usually marked by fatigue, hypoglycemia, low blood pressure, increased allergies as well as environmental and chemical sensitivities, estrogen dominance, and (ironically) poor wound healing—because your body doesn't have enough energy (literally, enough glucose) to perform all its functions efficiently.

Lack of sufficient cortisol (which, remember, is anti-inflammatory) also leaves you much more susceptible to allergies, both food and environmental. And it means you don't have enough energy reserves left over to do things like repair tissues, or help your organs of elimination (the gut, the liver, the kidneys, etc) to do their jobs. This can lead to poor wound healing, and chemical sensitivity, too.

Case Study:

Jennifer, a 36-year old mom of two, came to me with a sudden onslaught of food sensitivities presenting with bloating, alternating constipation and diarrhea, and rashes. Her symptoms began about six months earlier, right after she and her family had moved away from the town where she grew up because of her husband's job. Jennifer had a great support network in her hometown, and both her parents were there to help with the kids, and she was having a hard time adjusting.

Given the timing, I told her that most likely the stress lowered her body's threshold for inflammation. She probably had some reaction to those foods all along, but she never noticed before because her adrenal function was strong enough to keep them in check. Now that she was stressed, her ability to cope with inflammation was compromised. We did food allergy testing (and also environmental testing too, since allergies are cumulative and she had changed environments), but we also checked her adrenal function. Sure enough, adrenal function was quite low. Jennifer admitted that she'd had a stressful few years when her kids were young, leading up to the move, which probably set her up for the major adrenal hit she took when they finally left their support system.

We put her on a full protocol to support her adrenal function, and also took her off of the foods that were bothering her, supporting her gut with glutamine and probiotics. I also counseled her to find a community here, even though it would take some time to cultivate, and to schedule regular phone, Skype, or FaceTime "dates" with friends and family back home.

Six weeks later she felt much better: better energy, better mood, better sleep, and also restored digestion. She had also joined a church and felt hopeful that she would be able to plug in to a small group there.

Your adrenals also produce a hormone called aldosterone. Aldosterone causes the kidneys to reabsorb sodium and secrete potassium, and since water always follows sodium, your blood volume increases, which means your blood pressure increases. In the later stages of adrenal fatigue, though, it's more common to see low blood pressure. That's because the adrenals are not pumping out enough aldosterone, either. These people will feel the room go dark when they stand up too quickly, and it'll take a second for their vision to catch up to their heads, a situation called orthostatic hypotension.)

Your adrenals also produce a hormone called DHEA. This is the precursor for both the estrogens (estrone, estradiol, and estriol) and testosterone. It's a secondary source of estrogens for women (at least until menopause) and a primary source of testosterone for women. Likewise, DHEA is a secondary source of testosterone for men and a primary source of estrogen.

This is one reason why women who have been under a lot of stress in their pre-menopausal years have such a hard time in menopause: their adrenals are toast. They can't compensate. Menstruating women with adrenal fatigue will also have a lot of trouble with PMS, because at menses, sex hormones drop (that's what causes the shedding of the uterine lining). If you don't have enough DHEA to compensate for this, you'll probably have a lot of issues with PMS, too.

DHEA also counterbalances cortisol. While cortisol suppresses the immune system, thins the skin, and breaks down bone, DHEA bolsters and builds up all of these, encouraging tissue repair. (Testosterone is considered "anti-aging" for a reason.) While cortisol suppresses the thyroid, DHEA also revs up metabolism. So hypothyroidism secondary to adrenal fatigue will improve as cortisol drops and DHEA increases.

Adrenal Fatigue and Estrogen Dominance

Adrenal fatigue sets you up for estrogen dominance. This predisposes women to PMS (irritability, weepiness, anxiety, depression, mood swings); breast tenderness; severe menstrual cramping; heavy, prolonged bleeding (menorrhagia); spotting between cycles; thick clotting in blood; acne; hot flashes and night sweats; water retention; fibrocystic breasts; fibroids; migraines; and endometriosis. This is because all of the adrenal hormones have a common ancestor: cholesterol.

Cholesterol is also the precursor of pregnenolone and 17-OH-pregnenolone. Those hormones are the precursors of all of the sex hormones in your body. They are also the precursors of the adrenal hormones we just discussed.

Progesterone (the main hormone that counteracts estrogen) is a precursor in the adrenal glands for both cortisol and another adrenal hormone, aldosterone (the one responsible for blood pressure changes).

While estrogen encourages tissue proliferation (i.e. makes more of your endometrial lining, which can lead to heavy periods), progesterone does the opposite, nourishing the endometrial lining in case you get pregnant. It also counterbalances the estrogen dominance symptoms above, helping to lift the mood, restore libido, improve memory, assist with sleep, and protect against endometrial cancer.

Of the adrenal hormones, cortisol is the most important. Too much is a problem, but too little is disaster. If the body has to choose which of the steroid hormones to make, it'll pick cortisol every time. This means in times of high stress, when we need more cortisol to counterbalance adrenaline, our bodies will pass right on through the progesterone stage and make cortisol.

If you're not already in adrenal fatigue, you can avoid it by learning how to minimize the amount of stress that you cause yourself, and properly dealing with the unavoidable stressors that remain (see Chapters 14, 15, and 16).

If you are already in adrenal fatigue, learning new strategies to deal with your stress plays an integral part in reversing it.

The Effects of Stress on Allergies and Autoimmunity

Most allergens stimulate the release of inflammatory substances like histamine. Lack of sufficient cortisol due to adrenal fatigue (which, remember, is anti-inflammatory) means you can't naturally suppress these reactions. So while you may have always had a sensitivity to a particular substance (food or environmental), it's not until your body loses its ability to manufacture enough of the naturally anti-inflammatory cortisol—that is, when you're really stressed for a prolonged period of time—that you start to notice them.

Allergies are one step away from autoimmunity: in the former case, your immune system thinks a friend is a foe. In the latter, your immune system thinks that *you* are the foe.

When you're super stressed, you're likely to experience more allergies and/or autoimmune activity than you used to. But it's a catch-22: if you have allergies and autoantibodies, you've got inflammation. Inflammation stresses your adrenals, forcing them to produce more cortisol to counterbalance it. So even if you don't have adrenal fatigue to begin with, the longer you struggle with allergies and/or autoimmune disease, the more likely you are to develop adrenal fatigue as a result.

Reducing Stress Through Time Management

The first thing you can do to reduce the amount of stress in your life is to make a list of your goals. Separate them into personal and professional areas, and within each category, separate those into long and short term goals. Personal goals might be things like getting in shape, spiritual growth, spending time with family and friends, or learning an instrument. Professional goals might be (for a small business owner like myself) developing a marketing plan, or enforcing one that is already in place. Or it might be studying a new topic that will enhance your career options down the line, or keeping up with professional literature. You know how they say, "If you aim at nothing, you'll hit it every time?" The first step to reaching your goals is always to make them explicit.

Make a list of priorities for each day, and keep it short. If everything is a priority, then nothing is. A list, even one you have created yourself, keeps you from the moment-by-moment crisis of wondering which task to attend to first. If the priorities aren't immediately apparent to you, just pick something. Write it down, and stick to it. Cross off the tasks as you complete them, so that you can see that you're making progress.

Once you know what your priorities are, structure your time to attend to them. Time that isn't structured often ends up being wasted. Stick to one task at a time and complete it in bite-sized intervals. While attending to a task, it's important to do your best to prevent distractions. Close Facebook Messenger. Close your email. Close Slack, or any other application that interrupts you. If it's an option, turn off your phone. Structure time at regular intervals to check email and voicemail, and only do it during those allotted times.

I use a couple of tools for this. When I was in medical school, I used an Excel (or Numbers) spreadsheet with an ideal weekly schedule, in which I blocked off my required tasks, and then allocated the remaining time to work towards the goals outlined in step 1 (usually in 1-2 hour increments if I had them). Now, I primarily use my Google calendar for this, because there are always events that don't recur every week. Then I use my journal to write out to-do lists for each day the night before, as part of my wind-down routine. I always have more than a few items that I want to put on the list, though, and while too many tasks on the list creates overwhelm and sets me up for failure, I also don't want to forget about them. So now, I have my "Goals for Tomorrow" list, and my "Future Goals" list. (The latter can be as long as I like, and if I happen to have extra time the next day to tackle a few of them, awesome!)

Tools like this keep me focused so that I don't waste time, and they also force me to incorporate my personal goals into my routine. Otherwise I'd always find myself doing whatever seemed to be most important in the moment, and before I knew it, all my personal goals would fly right out the window.

Another tip that I find really helpful: get up early. There are a lot fewer distractions in the morning than there are later in the day. Usually nobody expects you to be anywhere or to do anything in particular early in the morning, which makes possible many of your personal goals which might otherwise never happen. I get up at least two hours before I have to leave for the day (before I have to *leave*, not before I have to *arrive*). That way I can wake up, work out, shower, make a healthy breakfast and lunch, spend time in prayer and reading my Bible, and (depending on the day) sometimes work towards a few other goals, like reading professional literature, writing fiction, or responding to personal emails.

It can be difficult to consistently accomplish all that you set into a day, so it is best to create a margin. I've learned this the hard way—if you have literally every moment scheduled with no buffer in between, that's a perfect recipe for stress, because in the real world, nothing ever goes quite the way we planned. Leave room for the accident on the freeway that slows traffic down. For the unanticipated phone call. For a friend to ask you for a favor. The proper ratio is about 80/20—schedule only 80% of your time, and leave 20% available for "life" to happen. If you start to notice that 80% creeping up to 90% or 95%, it might be time to reevaluate whether some of your current goals really need to happen now, or whether they might be better saved for a different season in your life.

Don't forget to schedule time for yourself every day, and guard it. Treat this time like an appointment. It's not negotiable. Try not to set too many expectations for this time, either, or it may become just another "task"—if you spend half an hour just staring at the wall at first, that's fine! The point is just to slow down. Eventually, you will fill the time with activities that you look forward to every day. Remember, it is your responsibility to take care of yourself—nobody is going to do it for you.

Ultimately you are the steward of your time, and it is never worth it to allow yourself to get out of peace. If that happens, the answer is not anti-anxiety medication so that you can maintain your unhealthy breakneck pace… it's to treat the cause!

Of course, it's not possible to remove all of the stressors in your life through time management. There will always be other issues that we have to deal with. For those other stressors, the best thing that we can do is just learn how to manage our stress by properly caring for ourselves physically, mentally, and spiritually.

Reducing Stress Through Lifestyle

One of the most important aspects of stress management is getting enough sleep. Adequate sleep contributes to overall well being, including but not limited to improved energy and greater emotional stability. Not only does sleep help to improve your memory (due to neuroplasticity, the process by which new information is consolidated in your brain during sleep), it also improves performance at whatever you do. This latter benefit is likely due to the fact that during waking hours, a byproduct of neuronal activity called adenosine builds up, leading to fatigue and exhaustion. (By the way, caffeine works by blocking the affects of adenosine... but only short term.) Sleep gives your body time to clear out the "debris," as it were, and make way for a new day.

Eating a healthy diet is also important. High sugar, high saturated fat, and nutrient deficiencies can all cause inflammation and a physiologic stress response in your body. Certain nutrients, especially B vitamins, are necessary for the production of neurotransmitters. However, B vitamins are found in dark leafy greens (not exactly a staple of the Standard American Diet) and whole grains (but not white flour, which has been stripped of nutrients). Not only does white flour lack B vitamins of its own, it actually depletes them during the process of digestion. On top of that, white flour and sugar both lead to a glucose spike and subsequent crash, which also sets you up for fatigue and irritability. So eat your complex carbs: veggies, fruit, and whole grains, along with plenty of protein and healthy fats.

Take a fish oil supplement. Essential Fatty Acids increase transmission of neurotransmitters, inhibit the death of brain cells, improve communication of cell membranes (which are sort of the "brains" of your cells), and decrease inflammation. Everybody needs to be taking fish oil. (Just make sure you get a good one—they're not all created equal. More on this in Part 2.)

Make time to exercise regularly. Exercise elevates your mood by releasing endorphins (the natural "high") and improves your metabolism. This is the most potent natural antidepressant out there! It induces production of neurotransmitters that elevate mood, and increases blood flow to both muscles and the brain. Increased blood flow also increases delivery of nutrients and oxygen to those tissues, and eliminates waste products faster than would happen at rest. (This is important because toxic accumulation can also cause a physiologic stress response.) If you don't have time to hit the gym for an hour every day, simply incorporate movement into your day at regular intervals.

It is also important to maintain a positive attitude as much as possible. Thoughts easily become habits—negative meditation (or worry) produces a negative attitude, and positive meditation does the opposite. Just like any other habit, it's difficult to break the tendency to think negatively at first, but it becomes easier with practice. Be selective about the ideas that you allow to influence your mind. As far as you are able, surround yourself with positive people and uplifting media (books, music, movies, and the like), and shut off those voices that are negative or harmful. It still may not be easy at first to change habits of negative thinking, but this will certainly help to set you up for success.

Practicing effective communication is another important way to manage stress. Many stressful events in our lives come about as a result of poor communication, leading to tension in relationships. Diffuse these situations at the outset as much as possible in order to avoid larger problems later on.

Remembering that leisure activities are an important part of your health and relaxation. Consider joining a social or volunteer group with similar interests to yours. Schedule time to get away for the weekend, to go on vacation, or to spend time with people you love.

Remember, too, that every human has a need to connect with others. One of the most powerful ways to reassure yourself that there's nothing "wrong with you" is to talk to others in a similar circumstance. That's one of the reasons that support groups work so well. The Bible says that we are designed to carry each other's burdens (although each is supposed to carry his own "load", Galatians 6:2-5), implication being that while a load is small enough that we can handle it ourselves, a burden is too large to shoulder alone. Helping, cooperative workplaces or groups promote positive emotions and interdependence, rather than codependence.

Despite all the work you do to keep yourself from becoming stressed, there will be times that stress creeps up on you. It is important to have a regular practice in place to help you relax.

Relaxation Techniques

There are many types of relaxation techniques available to you; I am going to share my favorites. They are highly effective mostly because they are easy to do and can be incorporated into your routine fairly simply. Notice that all of the techniques I present to you involve a shift in focus—that is the key.

Prayer is the ultimate relaxation technique. The idea that we are in control of our own lives is an illusion anyway. Prayer reminds us to place our focus not on the problem, but on the One who can lead us to the solution. Pray about your concerns, but then be still and listen. You might be surprised what you'll hear.

Meditation is the art of clearing your mind and focusing intently on a single image, phrase, or idea. Worry involves the constant focus on a negative thought or idea, while meditation is the intentional focus on a positive idea. For example, meditate on Bible verses that speak specifically to your circumstance. Instead of worry and fear, this helps you to begin to see the positive solution you hope for as you focus on these words. Hope then turns into faith as you choose to believe the verses upon which you are meditating.

Use guided imagery. When you worry, you are using your imagination to envision a negative outcome. Why not use the powerful tool of your mind in order to achieve the opposite effect? There are many terrific guided imagery CDs that can help you with this technique if you are not yet adept at creating powerful images on your own.

Develop a yoga practice. This form of slow, methodical stretching holds each pose long enough to release stored tension in the muscles that are forced to relax. It also emphasizes proper breathing.

Deep breathing is a quick way to bring your body into a parasympathetic (or a "not stressed") state. When muscles are tense, they seize up, inhibiting blood flow and oxygenation. Deep breathing provides more oxygen to your tissues, helping to release that tension. Breathe in and out to a count of five seconds each, expanding your stomach rather than your chest. This drops your diaphragm, fills your lungs to capacity, and slows your heart rate.

If none of the other techniques have completely done the trick, get a massage. Massage techniques force blood flow back into tense muscles, which both delivers oxygen and whisks away toxins that have stagnated in the tissues.

Severe Adrenal Fatigue

If your adrenal fatigue is severe (this can be determined by a salivary cortisol test, but you might already know by the severity of your symptoms), then you will probably need more than just lifestyle modifications in order to heal. Those are necessary, but likely insufficient by themselves.

At that point I'd recommend adaptogenic herbs, as these can help greatly with supporting your adrenal recovery. Some of my favorites are Rhodiola, Holy Basil, Avena Sativa, Schisandra, Maca, and Ashwaghanda. I also often add in B vitamins, particularly Vitamins B5 and B6, and Vitamin C, since these are all necessary for adequate adrenal function. In really severe cases I will also add in an adrenal glandular (an extract of porcine adrenal, pituitary and hypothalamic glands, hormone-free) to give the body the building blocks necessary to repair adrenal function. The most severe cases of adrenal fatigue I have seen sometimes require this level of support for nine months to a year, along with lifestyle interventions to help minimize stress.

Addison's Disease, or true Adrenal Insufficiency, is a potentially life threatening illness in which the adrenals no longer respond to the signals from the pituitary gland. Secondary Adrenal Insufficiency is similar, but in that case, it is the pituitary which does not respond to the signals from the hypothalamus. In either case, these conditions require diagnosis by an endocrinologist, and will require replacement of adrenal hormones (hydrocortisone, as well as fludrocort, the prescription version of aldosterone, and usually DHEA as well.) If you think this is a possibility, please ask your physician to send you for testing.

Adrenal Supplements	Purpose	Dosing
Gaia HPA Axis	This is my favorite combination of herbs for modulating adrenal function.	2 caps in the morning and 2 caps midday, if necessary (not after 2 pm, as these can be stimulating)
Phosphatidylserine (sunflower-based)	This is the best way I know of to lower a cortisol spike (determined by a salivary cortisol test).	This depends on when you have the spike, but what I see most often is a spike at night, in which case I dose 300 mg an hour before bedtime.
Dr Wilson's Adrenal C	A sustained release version of Vitamin C and its cofactors, critical to provide building blocks for adrenal hormone production	2 caps in the morning, all the way up to 2 caps three times daily (not after 2 pm)
Dr Wilson's Super Adrenal Stress Formula	A sustained release version of all the vitamins and minerals necessary for adrenal hormone production, including a whopping dose of necessary B vitamins	2 caps in the morning, all the way up to 2 caps three times daily (not after 2 pm)

Dr Wilson's Adrenal Rebuilder	The "kingpin" of the formula: a non-hormone containing glandular extract of the hypothalamus, pituitary, and adrenals. This helps to rebuild from the ground up, so that you don't have to stay on all the other supplements forever!	2 caps in the morning, all the way up to 2 caps three times daily
Dr Wilson's Herbal Adrenal Support Formula	Another combination of herbs for modulating adrenal function—these are my go-to for patients who don't like to swallow pills, or for those whose primary issue is more mood imbalance than energy deficits	1 dropperful 1-2 times daily in water
Rhodiola	For my more sensitive patients who don't respond well to herbal combinations, this is my go-to for mood and energy boosting and increased efficiency.	2 caps in the morning and 2 caps midday, if necessary (not after 2 pm, as these can be stimulating)

The Take-Home Message:

- **Get plenty of sleep.** Once you find your "sweet spot" of hours per evening, make sure you maintain an average of that number of hours every night. Go to bed before 11 pm if possible, as early evening is the most restorative sleep time for your adrenal recovery.

- **Manage your stress**. Find a stress management technique, or several, that work for you.
- **Eat clean, and keep your blood sugar stable**. A blood sugar roller coaster is toxic to your adrenal glands. Make sure you're having some protein every time you eat!
- **Structure your time.** Make sure you are in control of scheduling "you" time, and give yourself a buffer so that you aren't rushing from one activity to the next at breakneck speed.
- **Consider getting a salivary cortisol test** from your naturopathic physician or health care practitioner to see if you need extra support.

Chapter 6

PROLONGED POOR TREATMENT = HORMONES GONE HAYWIRE

The natural result of toxic living, bodily dysfunction, stress, and exhaustion is unbalanced hormones (particularly thyroid and sex hormones). Remember that everything is connected: the thyroid profoundly affects digestion. An under-functioning thyroid can lead to constipation, bloating, slowed bowel transit, and even SIBO. Many women develop bloating and constipation around their periods, or in peri- or post-menopause. Men and women alike develop blood sugar issues and weight gain with hormonal fluctuations, which certainly does lead to overgrowth of bad gut flora (see Chapter 4), and can also lead to SIBO. In short, hormonal problems are frequently the symptom that will finally send a patient to the doctor after they have ignored all the other warning signs.

Because hormonal problems can be tricky to deal with, let's cover exactly what causes them, how to test for them, and, most importantly, what to do to get back in balance.

Hypothyroidism

Your pituitary produces the hormone TSH (Thyroid Stimulating Hormone). It tells your thyroid (a gland that sits in front of your neck, right below your voice box) to produce the inactive thyroid hormone T4 (so called because it has four iodine atoms bound to it). T4 then travels to your peripheral tissues, where it gets converted to T3 (meaning it loses one iodine), and becomes active. The active hormone T3 is heavily involved in controlling your metabolism.

Clearly, an iodine deficiency will negatively impact the production of thyroid hormones, but that is not the *only* cause of hypothyroidism.

Tyrosine, selenium, zinc and a number of other necessary nutritional cofactors are used as building blocks to create active thyroid hormone. This is more likely the cause of hypothyroidism if the diet is especially poor, or there's some other malabsorption syndrome present.

Hashimoto's, or antibodies against the thyroid, is a very common cause of hypothyroidism. Autoimmunity in general has its own set of causality. However, production of thyroid hormone creates oxidative stress, which requires selenium for clean-up. Without this clean-up, autoimmunity can set in. So selenium deficiency may be one risk factor.

Hypothyroidism can also be caused by mercury toxicity. Heavy metals in general are bad news, but mercury particularly can antagonize selenium, which, as has been mentioned, is necessary for multiple steps of thyroid hormone production.

It is also possible to unintentionally suppress thyroid activity with prescription drugs. Amiodarone and lithium are two well-documented examples of thyroid suppressing drugs.

The tests for hypothyroidism are easy, but the interpretation is often far from straightforward. Most doctors will run labs for TSH only, or occasionally T4. Elevated TSH means that the thyroid isn't responding to the signal from the pituitary, so the pituitary effectively "shouts louder." Sometimes, though, the thyroid remains unresponsive. It is possible for TSH and total T4 to both be normal, while patients are still functionally hypothyroid.

Functional hypothyroidism can be caused by higher circulating TBG (thyroxine-binding globulin). T4 and T3 hormones that are bound to TBG are not available to stimulate receptors. This is a good reason to test free T4 and free T3, not just the total amounts of both. One possible cause for high TBG is estrogen dominance, which can also cause a host of female hormonal problems.[4]

A sluggish liver can also cause hypothyroidism. About 60% of your T4 gets converted to T3 in your liver… a process requiring selenium (again) and magnesium. If your liver is backed up (and one way to tell is if you have had a history of toxic exposure, and if you are chemically sensitive now), this might not happen efficiently. (Notice again how interconnected your body is!)

Functional hypothyroidism can sometimes occur because of a higher conversion of T4 to rT3 (reverse T3, which is inactive), instead of active T3. Your liver converts some T4 to rT3 when it has too much of the former, which, in the correct ratios, is a normal process. However, in times of high stress (read: high circulating cortisol), your body is in crisis mode. This means it needs to conserve energy to deal with the stressor, so things like growth and metabolism become a lot less important. If you're chronically stressed out all the time, this process might be ongoing (and it might also lead to leptin resistance, for patients who can't lose weight).

I mention functional hypothyroidism because many patients that have normal lab results have classic hypothyroid symptoms which are relieved by thyroid support or supplementation. Some symptoms to watch out for are sensitivity to cold, difficulty concentrating, constipation, depression, fatigue (and possibly weakness), heavy menstrual bleeding, joint/muscle pain, thinning eyebrows, brittle hair or fingernails, and unintentional weight gain. Most of my hypothyroidism patients also suffer from gut problems—perhaps just constipation and subsequent bloating, but often the slower gut motility can lead to dysbiosis and SIBO (Small Intestine Bacterial Overgrowth—see Chapter 4). Patients with Hashimoto's Thyroiditis often also have leaky gut syndrome (see Chapter 1) or gut inflammation secondary to toxic exposure (see Chapter 2).

You can support your thyroid by drinking filtered water, minimizing bread products, taking a high quality multivitamin and fish oil, buying wild-caught Pacific seafood, and minimizing stress. If you don't have adequate selenium in your diet, four brazil nuts daily will give you your daily dose. And, if you think that your sluggish thyroid is caused by toxicity, try a liver cleanse and consider having your mercury amalgams replaced (by a biological dentist who knows how to do it safely!)

If thyroid medication is required, I prefer to treat hypothyroidism with NatureThroid or Armour (glandular products containing T1, T2, T3, T4, and calcitonin, as well as the building blocks to repair the thyroid), since in my experience, most patients do much better on those than on Synthroid or Levothyroxine (T4 only). There is the occasional exception, though: I've had a few patients (maybe 5-10%) who have not responded to the natural thyroid at all, and who have required synthetic.

Halides and Your Thyroid

Halides are one of the classes of compounds that adversely affect our endocrine signaling system and are one of the possible causes of the epidemic of hypothyroidism. One major contender is toxic halogens (bromine and fluoride) which pop up in a number of places in our society.

Bromine, for example, is an antibacterial agent used in pools and hot tubs, an agricultural fumigant, and a fumigant for pests and termites. It is in brominated vegetable oils found in sodas and beverages, and it's still in some medications, particularly for asthma.

But probably most significantly, bromine is added to bread and bakery products as an anti-caking agent. Back in the 1960s, iodine was added to baking products instead of bromine for the same purpose. But because the therapeutic window for iodine is low, there was concern that this would disrupt thyroid function. Therefore it was replaced with bromine in the 1980s, and bromine continues to be used to this day.

Fluorine is found in the water supply in many areas, as well as in toothpastes. Most of us know (or think we know) that fluoride reduces the incidence of cavities; however, studies now suggest that fluoridation of the water makes no difference in rates of cavities.[1]

Iodine is a critical nutrient for thyroid function, and since it's primarily found in iodized salt, seafood, and seaweed, many of us don't get enough of it.

Because of the chemical similarity between iodine and its cousins bromine and fluorine, the latter two can mimic iodine in the body, binding to its receptors.

These other halides block the body's uptake of iodine, potentially leading to goiter and hypothyroidism.[2]

It is possible to test for urinary excretion levels of fluorine, bromine, and iodine. This can indicate how big a problem these halides may be for you.

Eating organic food helps to limit our halide exposure by avoiding those food crops that contain elevated levels of bromine due to fumigation.[3]

It is also best to limit bakery products. If you eat bread, do your best to make your own! Manufacturers are not required to list potassium bromate or brominated flour on the label. Or, my favorite bromine-free store-bought brand is sprouted, 100% whole grain Ezekiel bread.

You might consider a multivitamin that contains iodine, and/or consume seaweed, unless you have Hashimoto's Thyroiditis, in which case you will want to limit your iodine intake until your antibodies are negative (as iodine can worsen the disease). Iodine and other halides are at odds with one another, and supplementing with one can supplant the other. Because the therapeutic range is small and both too much or too little iodine can suppress the thyroid, at this point I prefer food sources or smaller amounts, like that found in a multivitamin.

Remember, also, to properly salt your food. There is good salt and bad salt; what you want is the iodized Celtic Sea Salt, added to taste, and not the highly manufactured high-sodium containing foods. But it's not just the iodine that will help supplant fluoride and bromide—it's also the chloride, as chloride is also in the halide family. For this reason, a low-salt diet is likely to exacerbate halide toxicity. If you are eating a whole foods diet, rather than prepackaged foods, feel free to salt your food with sea salt to taste, unless your doctor has specifically told you to avoid salt.

Finally, avoid fluoride and fluorine by filtering your water and choosing a fluoride-free toothpaste. Filtering your water will also reduce your exposure to chlorine, which is a highly carcinogenic halogen.

The Iodine/Hormone Connection

Iodine is a common nutritional deficiency not only because it is blocked by halides but also because it is hard to find in food.

Iodine is found in a low concentration in the soil. To some extent this is natural (as you get farther away from the ocean), but it is also partially due to farming practices that deplete the soil of many nutrients, of which iodine is one.

Also, the iodine added to table salt is generally a reduced form called iodide. Iodide works just fine for the thyroid, but not for the breasts, ovaries, or prostate. (And by the way, table salt isn't the healthiest choice of salt for you anyway. More on this in Chapter 10.)

Sufficient iodine intake is critically important for multiple hormonal pathways, but the body prioritizes the production of thyroid hormones when there is limited iodine intake.

Iodine is one of the key nutrients required for the formation of thyroid hormone, and for that reason, the thyroid requires more iodine than any other tissue in the body.

Because it needs it, it takes it: the thyroid "traps" iodine first, before any other tissue can get it. But if there's not enough iodine to go around, the thyroid will swell up to try to trap it more efficiently. This is called a goiter, and it used to be really common, before iodine was added to salt in parts of the country too far away from the sea to have much iodine in the soil.

But there are other tissues that require a lot of iodine: the breasts, the ovaries, and the prostate.

To understand the connection between iodine, the breasts, and the ovaries, it is necessary to first discuss the different types of estrogen. The three main types of estrogen are Estrone (called E1), Estradiol (called E2), and Estriol (called E3).

Estrone is found in fat cells, and can convert into estradiol or estriol. Estradiol is the strongest of the estrogens, and responsible for most of what we think of as "estrogenic" symptoms, both in PMS and in menopause. Under the wrong conditions, it can be metabolized into 16-Hydroxyestrogen (16-OH), which is carcinogenic (cancer-forming).

Estriol, however, has been shown to protect against estrogenic cancers, decreases the risk of fibrocystic changes in the breasts, and can even help women with estrogen-related weight changes to drop the extra pounds.

Why this is relevant: Iodine helps to maintain the estrogen balance in favor of estriol.

(There are other ways to increase estriol, too, by the way: one great one is to increase your intake of cruciferous veggies such as broccoli, cauliflower, cabbage, and brussels sprouts. Just make sure you wilt them first, or they may block uptake of iodine. Then you'll be working at cross purposes!)

As I mentioned, the best way to get iodine is from seaweed or a multivitamin. Not everybody needs iodine though, so get your levels checked before you start supplementing with large doses of it (what's in your multivitamin is probably fine. Or, if you use iodized sea salt, that will also be enough if you are not deficient). Also, again, get checked for antibodies against your thyroid, as iodine can make Hashimoto's worse if it is present.

Acne and Your Thyroid

Hypothyroidism and acne are two very common conditions I treat. Acne is usually a symptom of gut dysfunction. Common causes of acne include hormone imbalance, a backed up liver, elevated androgens (hormones in the testosterone family) sometimes due to PCOS, too-high sugar and insulin resistance, food allergies, dysbiosis, and occasionally low essential fatty acids.

But sometimes, acne can be a symptom of hypothyroidism.

One common correlate to hypothyroidism is elevated cholesterol. This is because when thyroid levels are low, the liver isn't filtering the cholesterol out of the bloodstream as quickly as it should—which means it won't be available to the body tissues that need cholesterol to form all the stuff cholesterol makes. The most important of these in this case is progesterone.

Why is this important? Progesterone facilitates the release of thyroid hormone from the thyroid gland, while estrogen blocks it (which is why estrogen dominance and hypothyroidism tend to coexist).

Adequate Vitamin A is also necessary for the formation of progesterone... but there's another reason why Vitamin A is important. The best known treatment for acne involves retinoid drugs, which are derivatives of Vitamin A. Vitamin A works by encouraging the regeneration of keratin in the skin (which is why it's also in most anti-aging formulas). Vitamin A is a fat-soluble vitamin, found in liver, meat, eggs, and dairy. Its water-soluble precursor, carotenoids, are found in red, yellow, and orange veggies.

However if your thyroid is sluggish, you won't be able to effectively convert carotenoids to Vitamin A, no matter how many carrots you eat. (And there's a feedback loop between the two: if you're low on Vitamin A, you won't be able to effectively convert T4 into the more active T3.)

You might have noticed that it's all interconnected: low thyroid function can cause acne. But so can a low-fat diet, since you'll be low in Vitamin A, and so can estrogen dominance (and low progesterone). But then, low progesterone and low Vitamin A can also exacerbate hypothyroidism, too. The best approach is to keep all these factors in balance. Balance your hormones, skip the low fat diets, and balance your thyroid.

Do be aware that while Vitamin A in high doses does treat acne, it's not a good idea to take high doses of it without supervision, as it is a fat-soluble vitamin and therefore possible to overdose. Vitamin A in high doses is also unsafe in pregnancy and should definitely be avoided. (Balanced thyroid and progesterone hormones and sufficient dietary fat, on the other hand, are all very good ideas in pregnancy!)

"Bound" vs "Free" Hormones

When balancing your thyroid (and sex hormones,) it is necessary to consider the ratio of bound hormones to free hormones.

Think of hormones as keys, and the hormone receptors as locks. When the key fits into the right doorknob, the door will open. But you don't always want the door to open—or at least you don't want too many doors to open all at the same time. The way your body gets around this is to put "sheaths" on most of the keys; that way, even if they come in contact with the right doorknob, they won't fit. The sheath is called a "binding globulin."

Different binding globulins are specific to different hormones. The Sex Hormone Binding Globulin (SHBG) binds androgens like testosterone, DHEA, and dihydrotestosterone, as well as estrogen. The Thyroid Binding Globulin (TBG) binds thyroid. The Corticosteroid Binding Globulin (CBG) binds progesterone, cortisol, and other corticosteroids.

Binding globulins matter because only those hormones that are not "sheathed" by a binding globulin are what we call "bioavailable": i.e. available to stimulate the receptors (unlock the doors).

This is why it's important to check, for instance "free" T3 and "free" T4 in a thyroid panel, not merely T3 and T4. It makes a difference how much hormone is actually unbound and bioavailable. This is also an important distinction for testosterone, since SHBG has a very high affinity for testosterone. A man can technically have a normal total testosterone level, but a low free testosterone level, which will still leave him with symptoms of low testosterone.

"Bound" hormones go up and down for a number of reasons.

SHBG decreases when androgens are high, such as testosterone and DHEA. This can happen from supplementation, or from conditions that cause them to spike, such as Polycystic Ovarian Syndrome (PCOS).

Hypothyroidism decreases SHBG as well, which may partially explain the correlation between hypothyroidism and other hormonal issues, such as PMS and menopausal symptoms. By the same token, high estrogen levels can increase the Thyroid Binding Globulin, leading to symptoms of hypothyroidism as well.

Obesity and excess insulin trigger lower SHBG, and low SHBG also seems to increase the incidence of diabetes. This is partly why losing weight, minimizing sugar and increasing exercise is so effective at hormone balancing. Conversely, very thin or anorexic women often do not get their periods anymore, possibly due to elevated SHBG.

You can test SHBG and TBG directly, and in some cases this is clinically useful. But the first step is to test the free, unbound forms of thyroid (T3 and T4). And of the sex hormones, it is especially helpful to test the free and total levels of testosterone in men.

Women with estrogen dominance symptoms or PCOS, on the other hand, would do well to increase SHBG with diet and lifestyle modifications.

DHEA: What It Does and Why You Care

As mentioned in the previous chapter, DHEA (Dehydroepiandrosterone) is one of three major cholesterol-based hormones produced by your adrenal glands (the other two being aldosterone, and cortisol.) DHEA is a precursor hormone for estrogen and testosterone in both men and women.

Aside from its role as a parent hormone, DHEA also counters the effects of too-high cortisol. While enough cortisol is necessary to maintain your energy and to counterbalance adrenaline, too much is a problem.

High cortisol encourages weight gain and metabolic syndrome by increasing blood sugar and inhibiting conversion of inactive to active thyroid hormone. DHEA encourages a faster metabolism. While cortisol suppresses the immune system, DHEA supports it. It can be very helpful in modulating autoimmunity and allergies. And while cortisol "breaks down," thinning the skin, breaking down bones and speeding aging, DHEA "builds up," protecting against these deleterious effects. For these reasons, DHEA has been considered an anti-aging hormone.

DHEA deficiencies happen, though, because in a competition against DHEA, cortisol wins. Of the adrenal hormones, cortisol is the most important. Too much is a problem, but too little is disaster. If the body has to choose which to make, it'll pick cortisol every time. As we age, this happens naturally; in our 70s we only produce about 5% as much DHEA as we produced at twenty. This may partly explain why one hallmark of aging involves using up the body's resources without building them back up again.

Your body may also favor cortisol, leading to a deficiency in DHEA, if you're experiencing adrenal fatigue. Because DHEA is the parent hormone for estrogen and testosterone, sufficient quantities are necessary for hormone balancing. This is one reason why women who have adrenal fatigue have such a hard time both with PMS and in menopause.

Case Study:

Jessica came to me with Ulcerative Proctitis, a version of Ulcerative Colitis affecting the rectum. She suffered from frequent painful diarrhea, several times per day, as well as mucus and blood in her stool. Her gastroenterologist wanted to put her on prednisone and biologic medication, but she was hopeful that there might be a natural approach.

We put her on the Specific Carbohydrate Diet, and she opted for food allergy testing as well. I tested her adrenal function, as an indication of her body's ability to handle inflammation, and sent her for basic labs —including DHEA. Part of this is because, while cortisol breaks down, DHEA builds up. Many autoimmune conditions respond positively to DHEA support, when it is deficient.

At Jessica's first follow up, her diarrhea had just barely stopped after being on the diet for three weeks. At that visit we also removed food allergens, supported her adrenals with adaptogenic herbs, and added in DHEA, since her level was incredibly low (it was 20. Most women feel better when it's 120 or higher!)

By the second follow up six weeks later, not only did Jessica's stools remain normal and well-formed, but she also noticed that her mood improved dramatically and she felt more energetic, too.

Because DHEA is a natural substance, it is unregulated by the FDA. It's available over the counter, but be careful with taking any hormones without having your levels checked first. For women, too much DHEA typically results in an overabundance of testosterone, which can lead to abnormal hair growth, acne, and irritability. It's also possible for DHEA to convert primarily to estrogen in some women, leading to estrogen dominance symptoms such as mood swings, water retention, and breast tenderness. Men who take more DHEA than necessary will most likely find that most of it converts to estrogen.

It's important to know where your DHEA is at to begin with, and to dose only as much as you need.

PCOS (Polycystic Ovarian Syndrome)

An overabundance of DHEA or other androgenic hormones (testosterone, androstenedione) and estrogen dominance are just two of the hormonal imbalances in women with PCOS (Polycystic Ovarian Syndrome).

Polycystic Ovarian Syndrome (literally, multiple ovarian cysts) presents with a few key signs and symptoms, though not all of them are present in every case.

Classically, being overweight is part of the picture, though about half of the women who have PCOS are not overweight. When patients are overweight, however, the syndrome is also associated with elevated blood sugar, insulin resistance (and downstream hypertension), or even Type 2 Diabetes.

Because of their problems with elevated androgens, women suffering from PCOS often have irregular menstrual periods and anovulatory cycles. Anovulation, of course, causes infertility, which is another hallmark symptom of PCOS. The androgens may also cause hirsuitism (abnormal hair growth) and acne.

Because PCOS is found both in heavier and thinner women, there may be multiple causes of the syndrome. However, estrogen dominance is always a problem in these women, often due to toxic exposures to endocrine disrupting chemicals such as phthalates, Bisphenol A, cadmium, and mercury. Arguably, insulin resistance may also be a cause: too much insulin decreases Sex Hormone Binding Globulin (SHBG), which leads to more circulating androgens.

Women diagnosed with PCOS tend to have labs that show an elevated ratio of LH:FSH (the hormones in your brain that tell your ovaries to produce estrogen), too-high androgens (usually testosterone, free and total, as well as DHEA, leading to acne and hirsuitism and suppressing ovulation). Insulin is also sometimes (but not always) elevated, and cholesterol can be elevated as well, as part of the metabolic syndrome picture. Many of these women also have gut problems like IBS or occasionally SIBO, secondary to high glucose. Or, they may have gut problems because their livers are backed up, leading to hormone imbalance and leaving them unable to process toxic exposures and more susceptible to food allergies. (Remember, everything really is connected!)

Diagnosis is a combination of symptoms, biochemical signs (those that show up on the labs), and imaging (an ultrasound showing multiple ovarian cysts), combined with exclusion of other possible causes.

Some of the traditional treatment options for PCOS include Metformin (a diabetes medication, for those women whose PCOS symptoms include metabolic syndrome) and birth control (to regulate LH:FSH production and suppress over-production of androgens). Metformin does work quite well, for women who can tolerate it without side effects. I don't prefer birth control as a treatment, though, because it merely suppresses the problem. As soon as you stop taking it, the LH:FSH ratio returns to where it was before, and you still have to treat the cause. (Plus, birth control can cause gut flora imbalances, as you read in Chapter 4.)

From a naturopathic standpoint, the treatment will look somewhat different depending on the woman's symptoms (for example, if she doesn't have metabolic syndrome then we won't be focusing on regulating blood sugar, and if she's clearly had a toxic exposure to endocrine-disrupting chemicals, then detox will be a big part of the protocol). But one treatment I almost always include is inositol.

Inositol is present in muscle tissue as myoinositol. Inositol regulates both FSH and TSH (thyroid stimulating hormone), and also plays a role in regulating insulin levels. I consider it to be an outstanding treatment based on some very impressive studies: In one study, women who received inositol versus those who received placebo demonstrated a higher ovulation rate (25% compared to 15%) and a shorter time to first ovulation (24.5 days compared to 40.5 days).[5] In another study, women in the group receiving inositol saw a significant decrease in serum testosterone (both free and total), plasma triglycerides, blood pressure, and insulin levels.[6] And in yet another study, researchers compared Metformin treatment with inositol, showing a significant increase in ovulation (65% compared to 50%) and in pregnancy (30% compared to 18.3%) in the group receiving inositol.[7] Even for women who do not want to get pregnant, this is good news: it means the body has restored its natural hormone balance. Another form of inositol, called D-chiro-inositol, is better for decreasing androgen production. Myoinositol is better for a metabolic syndrome picture, and it also helped to regulate the LH:FSH ratio.

The bottom line is that combined with appropriate protocols to address blood sugar, cholesterol, insulin levels, hypertension, and clinical symptoms of high androgens, there are definitely good treatment options out there for PCOS. Inositol is high on my list—in combination with a full protocol to balance estrogen dominance. I also always put these women on a diet protocol to help balance hormones, involving avoidance of high glycemic foods and sugar, minimizing caffeine, organic-only animal products to avoid all the added hormones, and high amounts of cruciferous veggies such as broccoli, cauliflower, cabbage, bok choy, and brussels sprouts.

PMS & Cramping

PCOS is not the only hormonal problem associated with estrogen dominance. PMS is usually correlated with a high ratio of estrogen to progesterone. Although both hormones decline dramatically leading up to a woman's period, if she has relatively more circulating estrogen than progesterone, she is probably going to have an unpleasant week or so.

Most of us associate PMS with mood swings and cramping, but many other symptoms such as bloating, changing bowel habits, insomnia, poor concentration, joint or muscle pain, fatigue, headaches and migraines, acne (especially around the chin and neck for many women), water retention, and weight gain may be related.

Many doctors will prescribe hormone-based birth control pills in an effort to treat PMS and regulate the menstrual cycle. These are often effective, and while many women do fine on them, there are some long-term consequences which should be kept in mind, such as increased risk of certain cancers and of stroke (especially for women over 35 who smoke), and also disruption of bowel flora (see Chapter 4), which can set you up for dysbiosis and IBS symptoms.

If your symptoms are mild, you may be able to control the cramping and muscle pain quite well with over the counter anti-inflammatory medications such as Advil or ibuprofen. Although these too have their side effects with continued long-term use, once in awhile I see no problem with them for most patients, aside from the fact that they don't address the reason the pain is there in the first place.

For water retention, your doctor may give you diuretics (to make you urinate more). They work, but again, they don't deal with the reason you're retaining water in the first place.

For severe PMS, you may be given antidepressants, which help not just with stabilizing mood, but also have been effective for reducing some of the other symptoms as well. Most likely this is because estrogen increases serotonin, and progesterone helps increase activity of the GABA receptor (a calming neurotransmitter); so antidepressants will bypass the hormonal trigger and just affect neurotransmitters directly. Common side effects for these include gut and stomach problems of all kinds, sexual side effects such as lowered libido, insomnia, and occasionally they can actually intensify feelings of depression.

Naturopathic treatments for PMS address the problem from several different angles.

For most conditions, as you might have noticed, I start with what you eat. The hormone balancing diet mentioned in the PCOS section applies here, too.

Exercise is also very important: studies show that women who exercise experience significantly fewer PMS symptoms.

I hope you realize by now that your hormones are all interconnected, so it's important to balance your thyroid if necessary in order to deal with PMS, as well.

I recommend liver and gut support, probably at the same time. You may have high levels of estrogen because "bad" bacteria in your gut keep it from getting eliminated, because a backed up liver can't do its job properly, or a combination of both (see Chapter 2). This is the reason why so many women who have gut problems also end up with hormonal problems.

In the meantime, to treat the symptoms, we'll add in good oils (which function very much like Advil and ibuprofen, but without suppression) in order to decrease inflammation. Many women may also find that acupuncture, chiropractic adjustments, or massage are very helpful for this. Magnesium can help loosen muscles, regulate hormones and bowels, and decrease fluid retention. There are also a number of botanical medications that work wonders for hormone balancing—one of my favorites is Chaste Tree, also known as Vitex.

Bioidentical Hormone Replacement Therapy (BHRT)

Hormone replacement therapy generally refers to estrogen, progesterone, testosterone, or any combination of the three. Usually hormonal replacement does not directly affect the gut, but it may help indirectly: for instance, progesterone helps to support the adrenals (as it is the direct precursor to cortisol), and adequate adrenal support is critical for helping to heal gut inflammation. Or in some cases, adding some estrogen and progesterone enables a woman to sleep, rather than getting awakened with hot flashes every few hours in the middle of the night... and adequate sleep is a prerequisite for absolutely anything to heal. For a man, testosterone therapy can enable him to finally break the vicious cycle of metabolic syndrome, which means blood sugar gets under control, and therefore gut flora as well.

So in many cases, bioidentical hormones may be an important piece to the puzzle of gut health.

Estrogen has receptors in just about every part of a woman's body and contributes to health of the urinary tract, bones and muscles, blood vessels, skin and vaginal tissue. But, there can be too much of a good thing: once again, estrogen dominance (relative to progesterone) leads to symptoms like PMS, changing bowel habits, bloating. mood swings, cramping, fluid retention, fibroids and heavy bleeding, low libido, elevated cholesterol and triglycerides.

Progesterone helps to prepare the uterine lining for implantation, and so it begins to rise just after ovulation. Progesterone and estrogen decline together throughout the second half of a woman's menstrual cycle, and if the two are in balance, the symptoms associated with estrogen dominance should not occur.

Women also produce testosterone—about 1/20 of the amount of testosterone that men produce. Testosterone contributes to healthy libido, a sense of well-being and vitality, and healthy bones and muscles. When a woman is estrogen dominant, she may be clinically deficient in testosterone even if her blood levels of total testosterone are normal, since estrogen produces a protein called Sex Hormone Binding Globulin (SHBG). This protein binds testosterone, rendering it unavailable to the cells for use. (Again, that's why it's useful to check not just total testosterone on blood tests, but free testosterone. This gives you a more complete clinical picture.)

Until July 2002, Premarin, Progestins, and Methyltestosterone were the standard estrogen, progesterone, and testosterone replacement treatments for menopausal symptoms. However, the Heart and Estrogen/progestin Replacement Study (HERS) and Women's Health Initiative (WHI) clinical trials illuminated the health risks associated with synthetic hormones. Bioidentical hormones, however, do not carry the same risks.

Premarin is an estrogen replacement drug prepared from pregnant horse urine. These are conjugated estrogens, and they are not biologically identical to those produced in the body—which means they do not follow normal human metabolic pathways. They are associated with vaginal bleeding, high blood pressure, blood clots, stroke, heart disease, nausea, vomiting, headaches, fluid retention, and they may increase the risk of estrogen receptor positive cancers.

Progestins are synthetic progesterone molecules which are less effective than bioidentical progesterone. They can also cause side effects such as abnormal menses or loss of menses, nausea, depression, weight changes, fluid retention, and insomnia.

Methyltestosterone is a synthetic analog of testosterone that puts added stress on the liver, and is correlated with liver damage and liver cancer. The body does not recognize it, so it is not possible to correlate clinical effects of methyltestosterone with blood levels of testosterone.

Bioidentical hormones are still prepared in a lab, but the molecules themselves are identical to those produced in the body (hence the name). I still don't always prescribe bioidentical hormones first for post-menopausal women—sometimes a healthy lifestyle and supplement regimen is all it takes to alleviate symptoms of estrogen dominance or menopause. For others, though, bioidentical hormone prescriptions will depend upon the individual's blood levels of each of the hormones, as well as her symptoms.

The bioidentical estrogen replacements are BiEst or TriEst. Remember there are three bioidentical estrogen molecules, called estrone (E1), estradiol (E2), and estriol (E3). Estrone is not active in the body—it simply converts into estradiol. Estradiol is the one that is most beneficial in alleviating symptoms, but it is also the one implicated in estrogen receptor positive cancers. There is some evidence that estriol is actually protective against these estrogen receptor positive cancers. For this reason, BiEst is a compounded formula of just estradiol (20%) and estriol (80%), while TriEst contains all three. TriEst is considered to be the safest for women with a family history of cancer, since it contains only 10% estradiol.

Bioidentical progesterone is prepared from extracts of wild yam or soybeans, these counterbalance estrogen dominance symptoms, help lift mood, restore libido (by counterbalancing estrogen), improve memory, assist with sleep, and protect against endometrial cancer. They may, however, alter the timing of the menstrual cycle for women who are still menstruating.

Unlike methyltestosterone, it is possible to correlate blood levels with clinical activity for bioidentical testosterone. I usually prescribe this only when both the symptoms and blood levels agree. Since testosterone is a controlled substance, women whose prescription includes testosterone must have blood levels checked every six months, as opposed to yearly for just estrogen and progesterone. It is possible to overdose on testosterone—symptoms of overdose include aggression and irritability, acne, and abnormal hair growth.

Low Testosterone and Metabolic Syndrome

Low Testosterone in younger men is increasingly common. Meanwhile, some 35% of the U.S. population suffers from metabolic syndrome, defined as high blood sugar (but pre-diabetic), excess weight around the waistline, hypertension, high cholesterol and/or high triglycerides.

It turns out that these two conditions are not only linked[8], but that each creates the conditions for the other.

Here's how it works.

Low Testosterone Leads To Metabolic Syndrome

Testosterone shifts the body's composition toward more muscle and less fat[9]. The opposite happens when testosterone is too low: the body shifts its composition in favor of fat storage, rather than muscle building.

There is also an inverse relationship between high cortisol (the stress hormone) and testosterone: as cortisol goes up, testosterone goes down. (In other words, if you're chronically stressed all the time, it can lower your testosterone levels.) High cortisol encourages metabolic syndrome all by itself, since one of its main jobs is keeping your blood sugar high enough to deal with the perceived stressor. Unused glucose has to get stored… and it gets stored as triglycerides, packaged into LDL, and shuttled out into the peripheral tissues, where it gets deposited as fat.

Physiologic doses of testosterone also increase the production of Nitric Oxide (a vasodilator) by the blood vessels[10]. This means adequate levels of testosterone help to maintain healthy blood pressure, and therefore low levels can contribute to hypertension.

One more chicken-or-egg problem: symptoms of low testosterone include depression and fatigue. If you're feeling low, it's hard to muster the motivation to work out and diet.

Metabolic Syndrome Leads to Low Testosterone

In normal physiology, the pituitary gland secretes the hormone LH, which signals the testes to make testosterone. But high glucose in the blood will lower LH secretion[5]. So effectively, high blood sugar (one of the characteristics of metabolic syndrome) means less LH, which means less testosterone.

Another characteristic of metabolic syndrome is excess weight, or more fat. Fat cells contain an enzyme called aromitase, which converts testosterone into estrogen. So the more weight you carry, the more your body will take the testosterone you *do* make and turn it into estrogen. Symptoms of low testosterone and of high estrogen levels in men are quite similar.

Hypothyroidism can cause weight gain and high cholesterol levels (characteristics of metabolic syndrome), too. How this is relevant: the active thyroid hormone, T3, combines with Vitamin A to produce the parent of testosterone (pregnenolone). Therefore, if your metabolic syndrome is secondary to hypothyroidism, you will lack the building blocks required to make testosterone.

What to Do About It

Physiologic testosterone therapy (gel or injections) can reverse metabolic syndrome.[6] (A word of caution here: in my experience, especially men who have metabolic syndrome require the addition of an aromitase inhibitor medication, at least one to several times per week, along with testosterone therapy. This prevents the sudden high dose of testosterone from converting into estrogen, and landing you back where you started.)

Metabolic syndrome and low testosterone are self-reinforcing. Testosterone therapy is one way to break the vicious cycle of low testosterone leading to metabolic syndrome (and perhaps gut flora disruption), leading to even lower testosterone.

How to (Naturally) Increase Testosterone Levels

Controlling for age and other factors, testosterone levels have declined across the population over the past two decades by about 20%. This means that a 50 year old man now will have 20% less testosterone than a similarly healthy 50 year old did in 1993.[7]

There has been much speculation regarding the cause of this decline. One of them involves environmental toxins. Many commonly used chemicals have an endocrine-disrupting effect (i.e. they screw up your hormones), including phthalates, parabens, diethanolamine, triethanolamine, monoethanolamine, and toluene, to name a few. (Go back and reread Chapter 2 if this resonates with you!)

Another possibility is the obsession with lowering cholesterol. Testosterone is a cholesterol-based hormone; you must have sufficient cholesterol in order to make it. Conventional wisdom tells us to avoid cholesterol, and very common cholesterol-lowering drugs (statins) stop the liver from producing cholesterol altogether, which means that everything chemically downstream doesn't get produced either. This includes bile salts (which help us digest fat—where we also get our fat soluble vitamins), vitamin D, healthy cell membranes (VITAL for your health), and steroid hormones (such as testosterone, estrogen, progesterone, and DHEA, among others). An estimated 32 million Americans are on statins, so this could certainly account for part of the testosterone decline.

There's also a great deal of debate surrounding phytoestrogens, such as soy. While there are numerous health benefits from the isoflavones in soy, probably everyone (not just men) should avoid GMO soy—which most of it is—just to be on the safe side.

The two most commonly known effects of testosterone are sexual virility and increased muscle mass, so this means that lower testosterone can also lead to sexual dysfunction and/or lowered muscle mass (with a corresponding increase in body fat). But as mentioned above, low testosterone can also manifest as depression, low bone mineral density, low energy, and anemia, in addition to symptoms of metabolic syndrome.

There are some simple things you can do to increase testosterone levels. They're the same things I try to get my patients to do for other reasons, but I've discovered that when I couch it in terms of testosterone levels, my male patients are a lot more likely to comply!

To make enough testosterone, you need to get enough sleep. Sleep helps you lose weight, decreases your stress levels, and increases the secretion of testosterone as well as Growth Hormone, both of which help to build and repair muscle mass.

It is also helpful to lose weight, as mentioned above. Losing weight does not mean eating a low fat diet, but a low sugar diet. As a cholesterol-based hormone, eating animal products (where cholesterol is found) actually boosts your testosterone levels. (Perhaps there's a reason why men stereotypically love steak! The caveat to this, though: make sure you're eating clean, grass-fed meat when at all possible. And increase your intake of healthy fats.)

In general, don't eat processed junk full of chemicals. Your liver has several jobs, but the most important is to detoxify foreign chemicals. If your liver is busy detoxing, it won't be able to perform its other jobs effectively, such as breaking down complex molecules (like estrogen) so they can be eliminated from your body, or breaking down fat (where aromitase is stored, converting testosterone to estrogen). It's also important to eat your serving of veggies, especially cruciferous veggies, as these are great for helping your liver perform more efficiently.

Nicotine and other additives in cigarettes actually decrease testosterone production.[8] That means you need to stop smoking!

Exercise can raise testosterone levels. Cardio is good, but resistance training (to build muscle) is better; training large muscles like your quadriceps and hamstrings is best of all for boosting testosterone. If you're already in pretty good shape, you should focus on muscle building (as opposed to toning), which involves higher weight and lower repetitions. If you're not already in good shape, start where you are and go from there.

Another helpful tip: chill out. Stress (particularly feeling trapped or helpless) decreases your testosterone levels. Pick a few stress management techniques that appeal to you, and give them a try.

And, to protect yourself from too many estrogens, avoid toxins—especially those in your toiletry items (see Chapter 2).

How Caffeine Affects Your Hormones

I'll be honest: I love coffee, and it definitely has its health benefits. Coffee consumption in moderation decreases the risk of many chronic diseases, as it is high in the antioxidant polyphenols and also helps to stabilize and regulate blood sugar. But especially if you're a woman with estrogen dominance issues or low libido, mounting evidence suggests that coffee consumption in excess of two cups per day may make it worse.

All foreign chemicals have to go through either your liver or your kidneys to get broken down into simple enough pieces to get eliminated. Your liver has lots of different "queues" (called cytochrome systems) for breaking stuff down. Each chemical has to go through its own particular queue before it can get out of the body. And, as we all know, the longer the line, the longer it takes to check out.

It just so happens that caffeine and estrogen share the same cytochrome system (CYP1A2).

The logical conclusion here is that excessive coffee consumption worsens estrogen dominance, because while your liver is dealing with caffeine, estrogen can't get eliminated fast enough at that proper time of the month… making PMS, cramping, acne, fibrocystic breasts and any number of menstrual-related symptoms worse.

As a matter of fact, a research study found that more than 100 mg of caffeine daily (a normal cup of coffee contains 95-200 mg) will increase circulating estrogen levels to some degree, but up to 500 mg daily (around 4-5 cups) will increase circulating estrogen levels by 70%![9]

Excessive coffee consumption does not just impact women though. As both men and women grow older, production of testosterone correspondingly declines. For men, obviously adequate testosterone levels are crucial. For women, testosterone is also important for maintaining libido, building muscle, and maintaining metabolism. But research shows that the more caffeine you consume, the lower your bioavailable testosterone levels will be.[10] This is because caffeine increases Sex Hormone Binding Globulin (SHBG), which will bind testosterone and prevent it from doing you any good.

One or a max of two cups of (caffeinated) coffee daily will help you to reap the antioxidant and blood sugar support benefits of coffee… but don't go over two, or you'll risk the potential damage of abusing your adrenal glands, as well as screwing up your sex hormones.

The Take-Home Message:
- Hypothyroidism can cause constipation, bloating, slow bowel transit, and can set you up for dysbiosis (Chapter 4). Even if your thyroid is within the lab limits, if you have symptoms of hypothyroidism, consider seeing your naturopathic or functional medicine doctor for evaluation and balancing.
- Avoid halides, toxic to your thyroid, by avoiding commercial bread products and drinking filtered water.
- To maintain a healthy balance of sex hormones, minimize sugar, caffeine, and choose only organic animal products. Eat plenty of cruciferous veggies, as these help your liver to maintain a healthy balance in your hormones. (But wilt them, don't eat them raw—raw cruciferous veggies can 1) block absorption of iodine, and 2) make you gassy!)
- Get plenty of exercise.
- Get plenty of sleep.
- If you suffer from acne, in addition to other gut balancing treatments, this might be a sign that your thyroid needs attention too.
- If you're a post-menopausal woman and you're having a hard time getting your hormones balanced with just these interventions, consider bioidentical replacement.
- If you're a man with metabolic syndrome and low testosterone and you're having a hard time breaking the cycle, consider seeing your Primary Care Physician about testosterone replacement.
- Ask your doctor to check DHEA, SHBG, and iodine in addition to your other hormone labs if your symptoms warrant.

Chapter 7

TOXIC THOUGHTS AND LIMITING BELIEFS

A lmost all of my patients with digestive health problems have some mental and emotional component to their physical issues. This needs to be addressed with the rest. Anxiety is probably most common, but I certainly do see depression enter in as well.

Over the years, I've come to realize that any kind of mental or emotional problem has its root in imbalance in one of four areas, or possibly a combination of a few of them: imbalance in the neurotransmitters, imbalance in the hormones, dysfunctional or toxic life circumstances, and/or dysfunctional or toxic thinking.

So far, we've primarily addressed physical problems. Neurotransmitters and hormones fall under this category—and to some degree, circumstances might as well (if the cause of anxiety and depression due to your health). We addressed possible stressful circumstances a bit in Chapter 5, and we will revisit how circumstances can affect our health in Chapters 14 through 16 as well.

In this chapter we're going to focus on the last one: toxic thinking. Thoughts have a physical structure in your brain, and they can trigger emotions, which set off a cascade of hormones that cause physiologic changes in your body. If you meditate on negative things ("I'm a failure, I will never succeed", "the universe is against me", "I will never get well", "I'm not responsible for the course of my life," etc), this will influence your words; your words will influence your choices; your choices become your actions; and your actions will determine many of your life circumstances.

Fair warning: it's hard to address this topic without getting a little bit spiritual. It's important to remember that we are not just bodies and minds: our spirits contribute to our overall health, also, and cannot be neglected. I am a Christian, and go back to the Bible as my foundational source of truth. If this does not resonate with you, I'd encourage you to still glean what you can from the principles in this chapter, as I think they will still apply. Truth is truth, after all!

The Bible often refers to the heart as the seat of emotions and also the part of us that generates thoughts and beliefs (Mark 2:8, Luke 5:22), and God tells us that we are to guard our hearts "above all else", for it is the "wellspring of life" (Prov 4:23).

But how do we do that?

Recognize that thoughts are real, physical things.
Your body has to translate a thought or idea into a real thing in order for it to be stored in your brain. Brain cells, or neurons, look like trees. Thoughts and memories get stored in these neurons, and as you accumulate more information, the tree sprouts more branches.

Fear and anger both trigger fight-or flight stress hormones, which, short term, can lead to sweating, shortness of breath and a rapid heart rate. Over time, however, chronically elevated stress hormones can lead to not only gut distress such as constipation and diarrhea, but also high blood pressure, high cholesterol, heart disease, diabetes, insomnia, sexual dysfunction, anxiety, immune dysfunction, depression, and even cancer.

Depression has a number of physical side effects, including a lower threshold for pain, chronic fatigue, decreased interest in sex, decreased appetite, and either insomnia or hypersomnia.

Anxiety, or worrying, can have effects very similar to chronic fear. Long-term effects include immune suppression, digestive disturbance, tense muscles, heart disease, and memory loss, in addition to those listed under fear and anger.

This is why your thoughts deserve attention—what you think about becomes a part of your brain, and sets off a cascade of physiological effects throughout your body. There's no such thing as "just a thought"! Solomon said, "As a man thinks in his heart, so is he" (Prov 23:7).

It's also true that a thought may keep you stuck, and prevent you from achieving your goals. If you believe you are *not* responsible for the things that *are* under your control, including your needs, your desires, and feelings, then you are lying to yourself. That lie can keep you from doing what you need to do in order to get those needs, desires, and feelings met.

So the next step is to identify your specific enemy: what is the lie, and how can you recognize it?

Become aware of what you're thinking about.

Stop and listen to your internal dialogue. What are you telling yourself? What kinds of emotions are you experiencing as a result of those internal statements? If you're frustrated about a particular situation you're in, listen to how you talk to yourself about that situation. Are you saying things like, "If only *that other person* would do (blank), then this would all work out?"

This might take practice. Sit down in a quiet space and stay there until your mind quiets down. Then ask yourself questions in order to follow a train of thought to its root.

A few examples:

* I feel (*an emotion: anger, fear, depression, anxiety, etc*). Why? Where does this emotion come from? How long has it been there?
* What is it that I am fearing?
* What is it that I am upset about? Is it really as important as I am perceiving it to be?
* What is it that I am thinking?

Continue to ask yourself "why" to the responses of each of these questions until you come up with a statement that involves only you; nobody else. These are the core issues that you can take to the next step. Some examples:

- I believe that I will only be loved if I am perfect or easy to deal with.
- I believe that I will fail at everything I do.
- I believe someone else or some other entity is responsible for making my life work out the way I want it to.

Sometimes it's helpful to know where these beliefs stem from, what event in our lives allowed these lies to take root, but sometimes it isn't necessary. You will most likely know when this is or is not important. If you feel you need an answer to this question, stick with it until you get one. Don't be afraid to seek professional help to unravel these questions if you need to—that's what counselors are there for!

Now, for the next step: the Bible tells us that we are to "demolish arguments and every pretension that sets itself up against the knowledge of God, and we take captive every thought to make it obedient to Christ" (2 Cor 10:5). This means we are *not* powerless to control the thoughts we think. We get to pick what we think about. Like wild animals, running through our yard, we can cage up our thoughts.

Accept or Reject Your Thoughts

Decide which thoughts to accept and which to reject based on whether they are 1) truth or a lie, and 2) helpful or harmful to you.

I make this distinction, because even a true thought may not be worth the real estate in your mind, if it is not "honorable, right, pure, lovely, of good repute, excellent, or worthy of praise," as Paul says in Philippians 4:8. Choose to accept only those thoughts that meet *both* criteria.

This is a conscious decision. When you identify a thought as being either a lie or harmful to your well-being, rebuke it out loud and break its authority over your life. Refuse to accept it. Thoughts become words; that's why Jesus said, "Out of the abundance of the heart, the mouth speaks" (Matt 12:34). The reverse is also true; what you confess with your mouth eventually makes its way into your heart (Romans 10:9).

Once you have done this, you must *rapidly* replace the negative thought with something positive (and true)—otherwise, you will eventually be overcome, and "the final condition of that man is worse than the first" (Matt 12:45).

Reprogram the toxic thought with the truth.

The Bible says: "Do not conform any longer to the pattern of this world, but be transformed by the renewing of your mind. Then you will be able to test and approve what God's will is—his good, pleasing, and perfect will" (Romans 12:2).

You renew your mind with the Word of God (Eph 6:17; 2 Tim 3:16). This means you must find the specific promises to counteract the particular lie you are believing. Speak the truth out loud.

- If you lack confidence, find the verses that tell you your identity in Christ.
- If you believe you are not loved, find the verses that say you are.
- If you believe you are being cheated or slighted, find verses that promise justice.
- If you struggle with finances, find verses that promise provision.
- If you struggle with illness, find verses that promise health.
- If you struggle with anxiety, focus on verses that promise comfort and peace.
- If you don't know what decision to make, focus on verses that promise direction.
- If you feel the world is against you, focus on verses that promise favor.
- If you struggle with fear, focus on verses that remind you of God's faithfulness and the fact that He is worthy of trust.
- If you deal with depression, focus on verses that promise you the joy of the Lord.
- If you feel impotent, focus on verses that promise power.
- If you feel threatened, focus on verses that promise safety.
- If you feel like a failure, focus on verses that promise success and victory.

All of these verses exist in scripture, and there are a lot of them. I recommend you scour the Bible for your own promises, because the verses you find on your own will mean the most to you. You value what you "pay" for, after all—and in this case, if you put in the effort to find your own verses, you will be much more likely to put in the effort to follow the steps and reprogram your mind. Because let's be honest—that's not easy.

If you're not a Christian, can you still use this process to your advantage? Yes. Scriptural principles work, no matter who you are... the trick will be getting yourself to believe what you are saying, if you don't have an underlying trust that the promise came from Someone you can rely upon. But the more you say something out loud, the more your subconscious mind begins to believe it. This is the concept behind affirmations of any kind.

As you begin to reprogram your mind with the Word of God, your faith will grow, because "Faith comes by hearing, and hearing by the Word of God" (Romans 10:17). But it won't happen overnight. The Word of God is like a seed (Matt 13:22-23), and seeds do not spring up immediately after they are planted. Rather, they come up "first the stalk, then the head, and then the full kernel in the head" (Mark 4:28). Because of this, realize that you will need to tell yourself the truth for some time before it begins to take root and grow. But it will bear fruit in time, and the fruit of the Spirit are the positive thoughts you want: "love, joy, peace, forbearance, kindness, goodness, faithfulness, gentleness, and self control" (Gal 5:22-23).

Every time a toxic thought encroaches in your life, repeat the steps above.

If it is a lie that you have already identified and rebuked, simply use the faith that you have cultivated to extinguish it (Eph 6:16). If it is a new lie, identify the lie, find the scriptures that counteract it and tell yourself the truth from the Word of God until the seed takes root in your heart, springs forth and bears fruit.

From personal experience, this works. When I first started my medical practice, with no idea how to grow a business and over $100K in school debt to pay back, I had maybe two patients per week if I was lucky. I wanted to use the skills I'd learned in school to touch the lives of others, but I had no idea how to do that. It was a terrifying time. But I fortunately knew these principles.

So here's what I did: I rehearsed my victories. I wrote out every time in my life that the situation looked impossible, and yet God came through. When I'd exhausted that, I wrote out every time in the lives of someone I knew that the situation looked impossible, and God came through. When I ran out of those, I went through the Old Testament and found every story I could when the situation looked impossible... and God came through.

Then I wrote out every verse in my little database that promised that God is the same, yesterday, today, and forever. He will not change.

I wrote out only the best verses (there were too many to write them all!) listing all the specific promises above: provision, success, victory, direction, blessings upon my hard work...

Then I wrote out James 1:2-4, which says, "Count it all joy, my brothers, when you meet trials of various kinds, for you know that the testing of your faith produces steadfastness. And let steadfastness have its full effect, that you may be perfect and complete, lacking in nothing." I praised God that my trials were performing that work in me.

When this was all done, it totaled around 17 pages in my journal at the time. Every time I caught myself beginning to panic, I pulled out my journal and reread those 17 pages, out loud. At first I had to do this almost five times per day. But eventually that went down to four times, and then three, and two, and one... and then I had it. I'd effectively reprogrammed my mind to believe and not doubt.

It wasn't quick, but I did eventually see the substance of my faith materialize. I was told it would take me over thirty years to repay my student loans when I was in school, and some of my colleagues told me they had resigned themselves to the fact that they would die still paying their loans. But faith and patience inherit promises... I paid mine off in five and a half years! God IS good!

Even better than that, in the process of growing my faith for this trial, I'd produced a step-by-step process that I could use in the next time of trial in my own life. I could also share it with patients for their own struggles, from which there appeared to be no way out.

Indeed, "the testing of our faith produces steadfastness," if we do not give up.

Part 2

BUILDING BLOCKS
FOR A HEALTHY GUT

Healthy Digestion

In Part One, we dealt with many things that can go wrong in the digestive process, and suggested ways to improve or reverse those malfunctions. The second half of this book is about giving your body the building blocks it needs in order to function in the way that it is designed. Remember that because everything is interconnected, the lack of any one of these elements can set you up for disease and dysfunction—in your gut, and beyond. The following is a short summary of how to maintain the digestive health you have finally obtained from following guidelines in Part 1. (In other words, if you don't have time to read the rest of Part Two, this is your cheat sheet!)

1) Avoid highly processed foods.

Eating processed food can cause a number of issues, one of which is nutrient deficiency (see Chapter 10)—since processing often involves stripping foods of their nutrients. For example, processed grains typically have been stripped of the fiber and nutrients in the hull, leaving nothing more than the "white" carbohydrate and the protein (gluten, if it's a gluten-containing grain). Both macronutrients and micronutrients are necessary for your body to function appropriately.

2) Consume plenty of raw foods.

A food is considered "raw" if it is not heated above 120 degrees, and includes raw milk (unpasteurized and non-homogenized), raw honey, raw cocoa, and raw fruits and veggies, as well as fermented foods such as raw cheese, raw yogurt, raw kefir, sourdough bread, sauerkraut, pickles, wine, fermented beets and carrots, and fermented apple cider. (Note that I am not talking about raw meat here!) Raw foods naturally contain enzymes, probiotics, vitamins, and minerals—which means they actually help you to digest them. But food processing, such as pasteurization, or even cooking, tends to destroy these things. Pasteurization involves heating foods to high temperatures in order to kill off bad bacteria. The problem is, in the process, all of the naturally occurring enzymes are destroyed, as well as all of the good bacteria, and a good percentage of the vitamins and minerals.

Therefore, the healthy individual whose gut can handle the extra fiber should shoot for around 50-80% raw food. Not only are raw foods more nutrient-dense, but they'll also take some of the strain off of your digestive system.

Again, this assumes that your gut is already healthy! Fermented foods are contraindicated for those with yeast overgrowth or histamine intolerance. Those with gut inflammation such as diverticulitis will need to avoid heavy fiber until they improve. Some raw foods can also make those with a less robust gut gassy. But *if* you've dealt with your obstacles to cure, this is a good rule to follow.

3) If organic food is available and affordable, buy it.

As mentioned in the micronutrient section (Chapter 10), foods grown in organic soil have a full complement of micronutrients, as well as their major macronutrients (nitrogen, potassium, and phosphorus). Not only will they pass their mineral richness on to you—but for the most part they are grown without pesticides. (This means fewer unrecognizable chemicals for your liver to detoxify—

we covered this in Chapter 2.) And in the case of the agriculture industry meat products, it means greater nutrient density, less indirect antibiotic or hormone exposure, and far more essential fatty acids, leading to less inflammation.

4) Take your probiotics.

Friendly bacteria protect you against bad bacteria, secrete acid to help you absorb nutrients, and break down any larger food particles that your hydrochloric acid, bile, and enzymes might have missed. Once upon a time, before modern preservation techniques, fermented condiments played a central role in our meals. These helped to replenish friendly bacteria on a regular basis. Back then, we weren't using over-the-counter acid-blocking medications (PPIs and H2 blockers), nor were we feeding antibiotics to the animals we ate on a regular basis—so the health-producing bacterial populations were most likely to thrive in our gut. Since few individuals have not been exposed to medications that alter their gut ecology, I generally recommend probiotics.

5) Drink half your body weight in ounces daily.

Dehydration is a common cause for constipation. You should drink more than half your body weight in ounces if you live in a dry climate, or if you sweat regularly.

6) Exercise.

A sedentary lifestyle is another common cause for constipation. When you exercise, the peristalsis in your gut responds, encouraging the undigested food to proceed down the gut pathway. Eventually you'll also increase your metabolism, which will translate to a quicker bowel transit time, too.

To help you determine which of the building blocks you need to focus on, I recommend you take the following quiz. This will serve as your roadmap through the rest of the book.

What Are The Building Blocks You Need?

1. Do you feel like you have a good grasp on what macronutrients (proteins, carbohydrates, and fats) are, and how to choose good ones? Y/N

2. Do you understand how to tell which micronutrients (vitamins, minerals) you are lacking? Y/N

3. Do you feel thirsty all the time? Y/N

4. Do you drink at least half your body weight in ounces daily, and feel well hydrated? Y/N

5. Do you spend, on average, 15 minutes in the sun and in fresh air every day? Y/N

6. Do you find yourself yawning frequently, or otherwise starved for oxygen? Y/N

7. Do you slouch, and/or spend a lot of your time sitting down? Y/N

8. Do you feel like you sleep well, and wake feeling refreshed? Y/N

9. Do you exercise regularly, including cardio, resistance training, and stretching? Y/N

10. Do you feel like you have a healthy balance of work and rest in your life? Y/N

11. Do you feel lonely, either with too few people in your life or not enough who truly know and accept you? Y/N

12. Are you happy and content with where you are in your life? Do you feel at peace most of the time? Y/N

Key:

EVERYONE: read Chapter 8

If no to 1: read Chapter 9

If no to 2: read Chapter 10

If yes to 3, 6, 7: read Chapter 11

If no to 4, 5: read Chapter 11

If no to 8: read Chapter 12

If no to 9: read Chapter 13

If no to 10: read Chapter 14

If no to 11: read Chapter 15

If no to 12: read Chapter 16

THE ESSENTIAL ROLE OF YOUR MICROBIOME

I've mentioned your microbiome in Part 1, but let's dive a bit deeper now. Your microbiome is the collective term for all the bacteria that populate your gut—all 100 trillion of them. Not only do the many species of bacteria vary from individual to individual, but the relative percentages of each type of bacteria vary as well. Even though your microbiome is not technically "you," it's so important to your body's function that it's been characterized as another organ.

Your microbiome acts like an army, protecting you against foreign invaders (pathogenic bacteria, parasites, etc). It also helps to educate your immune system about the difference between friend and foe, making it very important to mitigate against and prevent allergies and autoimmunity. It also helps you break down your food. For instance, recent studies show that raw cruciferous veggies and certain kinds of beans can make us gassy because we're just not eating them enough. Other cultures with much higher fiber diets don't have that problem. (Just like with everything else—use it or lose it.)

Different Diets Require Different Organisms

Three studies[1, 2, 3] compare indigenous diets (consisting primarily of veggies, tubers, legumes, and high-fiber grains) to Western diets (consisting primarily of poor quality animal fats, sugar, processed foods, and low fiber).

They discovered first that the distribution of bacteria in the microbiome differs based upon dietary consumption of the host (that's you!). Researchers believe that this finding suggests that diets that include fewer complex carbs (typical Western diets) do not sufficiently "feed" the bacteria that helps digest them.

Second, Western populations have a very high proportion of the bifidobacillus bacterial species in their microbiome, whereas the indigenous populations studied so far have none at all. Bifidobacillus comprises a chunk of the microbiome of nursing infants in all cultures, however—the assumption is that bifidobacillus is correlated with consumption of milk. Cultures that do not consume milk beyond infancy (and most don't) wouldn't require this organism to help break it down into adulthood.

Third, indigenous cultures have a much greater biodiversity in their microbiomes than do Westerners. This may be due to the lack of diversity in our diets, causing the microbiome to respond by becoming similarly narrow. Another possibility is the overwhelming use of antibiotics, not only among ourselves for minor ailments, but also in the agricultural industry. Once a relatively minor population of gut flora gets wiped out, it won't be able to rebound—as far as our little ecosystem is concerned, it's extinct.

They discovered that the indigenous populations tested had not just greater biodiversity, but also significantly more short-chain fatty acids (SCFA), which are produced by the microflora, than the Western populations. SCFA are the food for the large intestine, allowing it to repair itself.

Why does diversity in the microbiome matter? For the same reason you shouldn't marry your cousin: diversity creates a sort of checks-and-balances system that prevents a single genetic weakness from wreaking havoc. Less bacterial diversity leads to a more tenuous balance, and greater susceptibility to illness.

Your gut is the gateway to pathogenic illnesses, and to noninfectious gut disorders like allergies and autoimmunity (see Chapter 1). It's also the key to protecting against these ailments.

The Take-Home Message:
- Your microbiome is important. Keep it healthy and diverse by eating a variety of whole foods on a regular basis.
- Help to replenish it with a regular probiotic: at least 20 billion organisms, and a 50/50 ratio of the bacterial families bifidobacillus to lactobacillus.

Chapter 9

Building Block #1: Macronutrients

The goal of this chapter is to discuss the three macronutrients in detail: protein, carbohydrates, and fat. You need all of them for a healthy gut, and to be healthy in general; you just need the good forms of them, and not the highly processed forms. At the end of this chapter, you should understand how to tell the difference.

Fat

Contrary to popular belief, **fat is not bad.**

You need fat in your diet. For one thing, your brain is almost entirely made of fat, as are the sheaths around your nerve cells. Fat protects your internal organs, it's a great energy source, and it's necessary to absorb your fat soluble vitamins (A, E, D, and K). It's necessary for healthy cell membranes, so that good stuff (nutrients, oxygen, cell signals) can get in, and bad stuff (waste) can get out.

Without enough fat in your diet, you will likely feel fatigued, depressed, and more prone to illness, because many fats are highly antimicrobial.

Unfortunately, the "fat free" craze has led to near elimination of the good fats, instead replacing them with sugar and "bad fats."

Quick Chemistry Interlude:

Fats are made up primarily of carbon atoms bonded together. Each carbon can make four bonds. A *saturated fat* is one that is already bonded to as many hydrogens as it can hold. Like this.

$$\begin{array}{cccccccccc} H & H & H & H & H & H & H & H & H & H \\ | & | & | & | & | & | & | & | & | & | \\ C - & C = & C - & C - & C - & C = & C - & C - & C - & C \\ | & & & | & | & & & | & | & | \\ H & & & H & H & & & H & H & H \end{array}$$

An *unsaturated fat* is one that has space for more hydrogens. Like this.

$$\begin{array}{ccccccc} OH & H & & H & & H & OH \\ || & | & & | & & | & || \\ H - C - & C - & C = & C - & C = & C - & C - H \\ | & | & & | & & | & \\ H & H & & H & H \end{array}$$

Neither of these are inherently bad, but it's mostly the latter that can turn into bad forms of fat—specifically trans fats (see below). These have hydrogens on opposite sides of the carbon chain instead of on the same side. This is bad because these fats won't lay flat against each other, the way natural saturated fats do. If trans fats get into your cell membranes, it means signals don't get in and out of the cells very efficiently. It also means nutrients and oxygen can't get in easily, nor can metabolic waste get out—leading to a buildup of cellular waste products.

Unhealthy Fats

1. **Trans fats, aka Partially Hydrogenated Oils.** In 1907, Proctor & Gamble devised the process of hydrogenation of plant oils in order to render them solid at room temperatures.[1] *Hydrogenation* means bombarding the unsaturated (liquid) fat with hydrogen ions to make it saturated. This process ended up creating trans fats, which are associated with most of the inflammatory diseases of Western culture (such as diabetes, heart disease, autoimmune conditions, allergies, and cancer).

   Trans fats are found in margarine, shortening, processed and fried foods of all kinds.

2. **Polyunsaturated vegetable oils.** These are commonly used in processed and fast foods, at which point they become trans fats, under conditions of pressure and high heat.

Many vegetable oils are omega-6 essential fatty acids, which are necessary in moderation. The ideal ratio of omega-6 to omega-3 essential fatty acids should be about 4-6:1, in favor of omega-6. But in the Standard American Diet, the ratio is more like 20:1. (Yikes!)

Why this is a problem: if you get just enough omega-6, you'll produce an anti-inflammatory molecule (called a prostaglandin). If you get too much, you'll flood the biochemical pathway and produce an inflammatory prostaglandin, which leads to pain—in fact, the inflammatory prostaglandin produced with too much omega-6 is the very chemical suppressed by aspirin.

In other words, inflammatory pain may be caused by eating too much omega-6 (mostly from vegetable oil and processed foods) and too little omega-3.

So if you avoid omega-6 polyunsaturated vegetable oils, chances are you'll consume enough in other foods to maintain an appropriate ratio with omega-3 fatty acids.

Polyunsaturated vegetable oils to avoid include: canola oil, corn oil, cottonseed oil, safflower and sunflower oil.

Healthy Fats

1. **Saturated Fats.** Too much saturated fat leads to inflammation. But too little saturated fat means too few essential fatty acids (see #3

below). If you eat saturated fat in moderation, you reap the benefits, and your body can convert the excess to essential fatty acids if it needs them. Saturated fat makes up 50% of your cell membranes (and healthy cell membranes means good stuff can in, and bad stuff can get out). They are also the preferred food for your heart, are antimicrobial, support immune function, are necessary for your blood to clot and for your lungs to work properly, are easily absorbed for quick energy, and are necessary for infant brain development.

You should avoid the saturated fat that comes from agriculture industry meats. Animals fed on their natural free-range diets have a 50/50 ratio of saturated fat to essential fatty acids. Fat from typical grain-fed animals is almost 100% saturated. This can lead to inflammation due to the deficiency in essential fatty acids (more on this when we discuss protein.)

The saturated fats you should consume are found in coconut oil, avocados, nuts, butter, ghee, palm oil, animal fats (grass fed and/or free range) and eggs (free range).

2. **Monounsaturated Fats.** Remember the picture of saturated versus unsaturated fats? Monounsaturated fats have only a single double bond in the chain. These are known to lower inflammatory omega 6, lower cholesterol and blood pressure, and maintain healthy nerve function. The most famous monounsaturated fat is olive oil—just look for "organic" and "extra virgin" varieties. This means it's unprocessed, and therefore still high in antioxidants.

3. **Polyunsaturated Essential Fatty Acids (EFAs):** these are the most beneficial type of fat, mostly because the typical Western diet is deficient in them. They're anti-inflammatory, support the mucus lining in your stomach, lower blood pressure and cholesterol, improve insulin sensitivity, decrease allergic responses, keep cell walls healthy, and are necessary for brain development.

EFAs are found in vegetable oils (such as flax seed and hemp seed), nut oils (macadamia, peanut), plant oils (pumpkin seed, grape seed, sesame, rice bran, borage, black currant, evening primrose), grass fed meat and dairy, and fish or marine oils.

One more thing before I leave the topic of fats...

A Word On Cholesterol

Cholesterol is not one of the major macronutrients; it's a carrier for fat. Fat gets stored as triglycerides, and triglycerides get packaged into either HDL (High Density Lipoproteins) or LDL (Low Density Lipoproteins), depending on whether they're headed to your liver to get broken down and used as energy, or whether they're headed from your liver to the rest of you to get stored as fat (respectively).

Despite its reputation for causing heart disease (which is misplaced), adequate levels of cholesterol are quite important, because cholesterol is a precursor for other things you need.

Just like saturated fats and essential fatty acids, cholesterol is necessary for healthy cell membranes. If your cell membranes aren't healthy, you won't be able to effectively let nutrients, oxygen, and glucose in, let waste out, or facilitate intracellular communication.

Cholesterol is also the precursor for estrogen, progesterone, testosterone, and all of the hormones produced by your adrenal glands, including DHEA, cortisol, and aldosterone. If you're a man, you definitely want to have plenty of testosterone (refer to Chapter 6). If you're a woman, you definitely want to have sufficient estrogen and progesterone, especially if you're peri- or post-menopausal.

Adequate cholesterol is necessary to produce Vitamin D. The active form of it comes from sunlight, of course, but you still have to have enough cholesterol in order to make it. Lack of vitamin D can lead to poor immune function, poor calcium absorption, and depression. I'll discuss more on this in the next chapter.

Cholesterol is the precursor for bile, which is necessary to absorb fat. If you don't have enough bile, then you're going to have trouble with fatty foods, and you won't be able to absorb fat-soluble vitamins either (A, D, E, and K).

Early signs of too-low cholesterol are depression, poor concentration and memory, and lower energy.

My Conclusion on Fat:

Avoid trans fats or high omega-6 fatty acids. Do consume good fats, including saturated fats from natural, organic sources, monounsaturated and polyunsaturated omega-3 fatty acids.

Also, be sure you're choosing the right fats for the right kinds of cooking. Even some healthy fats will go rancid with high heat, forming free radicals, while others are relatively stable. For this reason, you should choose different fat sources depending on your purpose.

For high heat cooking, use animal fats, butter or ghee, coconut oil, or palm oil.

For light cooking, use olive oil, avocado oil, macadamia nut, peanut, sesame, or rice bran oil.

For dressings: use flax, grape seed, olive, hemp, or pumpkin oils.

Protein

All of your cells are made up of proteins. Protein, in turn, is made up of amino acids (twenty of them, to be exact). Your DNA codes for each one of those individual amino acids and, like beads on a chain, your cells assemble the amino acids in sequence such that proteins can be formed. Your body is capable of forming some of those amino acids on its own, but there are others, called essential amino acids, which you have to ingest from your diet. If you don't, you will be malnourished—meaning your body will not be able to perform some of its essential functions.

The most abundant sources of protein are meat and animal products, such as eggs, cheese, and dairy. Fish and seafood fall under this category too. Vegetarian sources include beans, tofu, nuts, and seeds.

This is a good place to cover the question that generally comes up in this category, and that is this: *aren't vegetarian sources of protein healthier than animal-based sources?*

The China Study was the source of this argument. The most comprehensive study in nutrition ever conducted, it spanned 65 counties in China and resulted in over 8000 statistically significant associations between diet, lifestyle, and disease.[2] They compared the plant-based rural diets in certain parts of China to the Americanized Western diet, which includes high amounts of meat. Not surprisingly, they found that Westernized parts of China experienced far higher incidences of Western diseases of affluence (including cardiovascular disease, diabetes, autoimmune disease, and cancer), compared to those parts of China still consuming their whole food, plant-based fare.

The conclusion was that increased meat intake is responsible for the Western diseases of affluence.

The problem with this reasoning is that correlation does not equal causation. Our earlier generations enjoyed meat without experiencing the explosion of health issues we see today. An alternate cause of our current state of poor health rests with the methods employed by the Western agriculture industry.

What's So Bad about Agriculture Industry Animal Products?

Feedlots are designed to make a profit, like any business. The more animals that are raised and slaughtered in a given amount of time, the more profitable the business. In order to maximize this turnover, however, conditions for the animals are poor... which is bad news, even if you are not an animal activist. Because infection is rampant, dairy cows alone consume about 70% of the nation's antibiotics, contributing to the problem of antibiotic-resistant bacteria.[3]

Those animals fattened up for slaughter are fed grain (mostly corn) instead of grass. Cattle stomachs are not designed to digest corn. This leads to a weakened immune system and increased susceptibility to infection, increasing the need for prophylactic antibiotics (thus speeding development of antibiotic resistant bacteria even more). Also, animals that consume corn instead of grass produce meat whose fat is completely saturated, compared to the 50/50 ratio of saturated to polyunsaturated fats produced by grass-fed animals. Again, some saturated fat is necessary, but excess can lead to a relative deficiency of essential fatty acids, and inflammation.

If that wasn't enough, the corn these animals consume is genetically modified... and the evidence suggests that GMO foods lower the animals' nutrient absorption.[4] When we, in turn, eat the meat from these animals, this lower nutrient content gets passed along to us.

What's So Good about Organic and Grass-Fed Meat?

Organic, grass-fed animals are allowed to roam free (at least in theory—this isn't well regulated) and consume their natural diet of grass. As a result, not only is the treatment of the animals significantly more humane, but the fat in the meat is about a 50/50 ratio of saturated fats to anti-inflammatory and heart healthy essential fatty acids; the nutrient content of the meat remains intact; and the necessity for antibiotics dramatically declines.

Additionally, adding meat and animal products to your diet provides a much more substantial serving of protein than most plant-based protein sources can provide.

Vegetarian Proteins

If you choose to avoid animal products, the main nutrients you will need to monitor and possibly replace are iron and B12, which are found primarily in meat. The lack of either or both of these can contribute to fatigue, and potentially other deficiency symptoms as well (more on specific nutrient deficiencies in Chapter 10).

If you're a vegetarian, you will need to be vigilant about your protein intake, as you need adequate protein and fats to prevent the blood sugar roller coaster from a diet comprised primarily of carbohydrates, and to keep your gut flora balanced.

Case Study:

Laine was a 25-year old world traveler, who came to me in between trips with constant gas and bloating, brain fog, and fatigue. She was vegan, and proud of her healthy, whole-foods-based diet. However, her diet diary showed that as a result, she consumed mostly grains and fruit, with occasional vegetables. Every now and then she added in nuts or tofu, but inconsistently at best. While she did a great job of choosing nutrient-dense foods, the lack of protein caused the comparatively simple carbs in grains and fruit to hit her bloodstream quickly, feeding the population of candida (a fungal organism, see

Chapter 4) in her gut. As a byproduct, these candida produced gas, and caused her other symptoms.

Once we restricted all simple carbs, killed off the organisms, repopulated with good gut flora, and added a form of protein with every meal, Laine's symptoms resolved.

Historically vegetarians relied on soy as a protein staple, but soy has been vilified and thus is falling out of favor. Men avoid it out of fear that it may cause them to develop breast tissue, also known as gynecomastia. Women avoid it out of fear that it may throw their already precarious thyroid numbers out of balance, or that it may increase the risk of hormone-based cancers. I'll address the thyroid and phytoestrogen issues separately.

Phytoestrogens are 100 to 1000 times weaker than the estrogen your body produces naturally. What this means: both types of molecules bind to estrogen receptors the same way a key might fit into a lock—but the resulting effects of this match will be very different. If you have too few natural estrogen molecules in your body, such as in menopause, phytoestrogens will bind to your estrogenic receptors and weakly stimulate them, which may help improve symptoms of too little estrogen. If you have too much estrogen relative to progesterone, however (such as in endometriosis, PMS, some menstrual migraines, etc), then a phytoestrogen will still stimulate that estrogen receptor, but it will do so 100 to 1000 times less than the estrogen molecule that otherwise would have occupied that spot. In other words, phytoestrogens can be either estrogenic *or* anti-estrogenic, depending on which one your body needs.

So I wouldn't worry about soy just because it's a phytoestrogen, unless you have a personal history of an estrogen receptor positive cancer, and you are carefully avoiding *all* estrogenic stimulation.

Case Study:

Maria came to me when she was 48, post-menopause, with fatigue, hot flashes, night sweats, mood swings, and headaches. She'd gotten much worse when her Primary Care Physician prescribed estrogen for her symptoms, and she came to me looking for alternatives. My assessment was that, while her hormones were all quite low, her estrogen was relatively higher than her progesterone levels.

She did not want to take progesterone, having been a bit "snake-bit" with hormones already. So instead I put her on a diet eliminating sugar, white carbohydrates, and caffeine, increasing cruciferous veggies, and increasing her non-GMO soy intake. This turned out to be all she needed: a diet that helped her liver to eliminate excess estrogen, combined with a regular dose of soy balanced her hormones well enough that her symptoms disappeared.

The connection between soy and thyroid suppression has nothing to do with its status as a phytoestrogen. Several other foods considered to be thyroid suppressants (aka *goitrogens*) include millet, peanuts, radishes, turnips, and raw cruciferous veggies (such as cauliflower, brussels sprouts, and broccoli). These are very healthy foods overall, and it would be a mistake to completely avoid them. Goitrogens are only a problem for thyroid function if you're already iodine deficient. Iodine is one of the minerals necessary for the formation of thyroid hormone, and goitrogens compete with thyroid hormone for iodine. So as long as your iodine status is not a problem, you need not avoid these foods—including soy. Even if you *are* iodine deficient (which isn't uncommon—I run blood tests for this regularly), fermenting, cooking, or steaming these goitrogens renders them safe for consumption. Fermented soy products include natto, miso, soy sauce, and tempeh.

However (and this is a big however), soy is one of the foods that is most commonly genetically modified—we're talking 94% of the soy in the U.S. It still isn't absolutely clear what effects genetic modification may have on health, but because there is plenty of evidence to suggest there might be a problem, I choose to play it safe and avoid GMO soy (we discussed this more in chapter 1).

The other major plant-based protein source, beans, contain carbohydrates that are difficult to break down, which can contribute to gas and bloating. For this reason, my vegetarian and vegan patients whose guts are not especially robust tend to have a harder time consuming adequate protein.

High Protein Fad Diets

You don't want to emphasize protein too much either, contrary to such fad diets as South Beach, Atkins, and Bernstein. While these diets will lower cholesterol, triglycerides, insulin resistance, and weight, *too much* protein over a period of time can lead to kidney damage, weight loss, and (depending on the type of protein consumed) high saturated fat relative to essential fatty acids. It can also set you up for nutrient deficiencies if your primary source of nutrition is meat. Also, your body runs on glucose from carbohydrates, not protein—so although it is possible for your body to turn protein into energy, it's not nearly as efficient, so you may feel exhausted. And finally, the lack of fiber inherent in high protein diets may lead to constipation.

Case Study:

Jeff came to me with bloating and constipation with almost any carbohydrate he put into his mouth. He'd learned to deal with this by eating almost exclusively protein. I frowned when I saw this, and asked to see his most recent blood work to check his kidneys. He told me he hadn't brought it, but that doctors in the past had told him he had kidney problems. He also said he could not drink enough water to stay hydrated.

I sent him home with a stool culture, suspecting candida and possibly some other dysbiotic organism causing the symptoms, and also recommended electrolytes and the amino acid taurine to assist with his absorption of fluids. While we waited for the results, I recommended that he restrict protein to no more than 30% of his diet, and add in fish oil for further kidney protection.

Jeff's test results came back positive for candida, and also two other pathogenic bacteria. At the next visit he said he was hydrating much better. I put him on a diet and supplement protocol for six weeks, and sent him home with a requisition to re-check his kidneys.

Six weeks later, his bloating and constipation with carbs was resolved, and kidney function had returned to normal on lab work.

My Conclusion on Protein:

For most healthy patients, I encourage organic or free-range animal protein consumption as part of a balanced, whole-foods diet, except for those who abstain for religious or ethical reasons. There are certain conditions which do require avoiding animal proteins for a period of time, though.

And I will say this: If your choice is between whole food vegetarianism or veganism and the Standard American Diet, there's no doubt that the former is healthier!

Carbohydrates ("Carbs")

As previously mentioned, carbohydrates are the macronutrient most efficiently turned into glucose, which is your body's primary fuel source. The more complex the carbohydrates are (i.e. the bigger the molecule), the more work your body has to do in order to release its energy potential. Another way to say this is that complex carbs have a lower glycemic index.

The glycemic index is a measure of how quickly a particular food turns to sugar in the body. Glucose is assigned a glycemic index of 100, and everything else is assigned a number relative to that. At the top of the glycemic index list are all things white, especially processed white flour (including white bread, pancakes, and pastries), most processed white grains (including white rice, instant oatmeal, popcorn, and most cereals), and white potatoes, especially potato products (including french fries, potato chips, and instant mashed potatoes). The most complex carbohydrates, those with the lowest glycemic index, are generally vegetables (starchy ones excepted), followed by fruit and whole grains.

Sugar tastes good to us because it's a source of quick energy, which historically was a lot more scarce than it is today. It can get converted into ATP, the currency your body uses for energy, very quickly. But your blood can only accommodate a few tablespoons of sugar at a time.

Picture table sugar—it's granular and it has relatively rough edges. If you have too much sugar in your bloodstream over a period of time, those rough edges nick the walls of your blood vessels and cause damage. When that happens, your body has to patch up the damage with a "bandage," so that it can heal.

The "bandage" is called LDL (aka "bad" cholesterol). The more extensive the damage, the more cholesterol you need to form an adequate band-aid. But with continued high intake of sugar, over time that LDL plug gets bigger and bigger. Eventually it may impede blood flow, or the plug can become unstable and break off, traveling to some other part of the body until it encounters a blood vessel too small to accommodate it. (This is cardiovascular disease—and it can lead to heart attacks and strokes.) **Cardiovascular disease is problem #1 with too much sugar.** (Note that the LDL was *not* the culprit—it only showed up to try to fix the problem!)

Your body tries to get rid of excess sugar from the bloodstream in order to minimize this process. Sugar has to get inside the cells in order to get out of the blood. Sugar can't just rush into the cells directly though—it has to have the "key" to get in. The key is insulin, which is produced by the pancreas in response to high sugar in the bloodstream. This works great for awhile... but problems arise when this cycle is repeated too often, too long. Like a drug addict needing a bigger dose to achieve the same high, the body will start to require more and more insulin to keep up with your sugar intake. Eventually, the pancreas can't keep up with the demand. This leads to **Insulin Resistance and Diabetes, problem #2 with too much sugar.**

Once the sugar gets inside the cells, it can't be stored in its present form—it has to be converted from "quick" energy into "potential" energy—aka fat (or more precisely, triglycerides.) So excess sugar also leads to obesity. **Obesity is problem #3 with too much sugar.**

There are even more potential issues than this. But for now, suffice it to say that too much sugar is no small part of the epidemic of obesity, diabetes, and cardiovascular disease in this nation. The average American consumes about 156 pounds of it per year![5]

My Conclusions on Carbohydrates

The best carbs are veggies, hands down. They are super nutrient dense, and full of fiber that will help to keep your gut healthy and eliminate toxins. A healthy diet will also include 100% whole (i.e. unprocessed) grains and a variety of different types of fruits—the more colorful the better.

You don't want a diet that's primarily complex carbs to the exclusion of adequate fat and protein, though. High carb fad diets such as Ornish, Pritikin, McDougall, and Swank Diets will lead to lower cholesterol and triglycerides, weight loss, lower cardiovascular and cancer risk, and a healthier gut due to the high fiber. However, they can set you up for deficiencies in essential fatty acids (since those are fat), and in fat-soluble vitamins (A, D, E, and K). Some people also feel inordinately hungry on a high carb diet, and potentially hypoglycemic.

Do minimize sugar and simple carbs as much as you can. Make them an occasional treat, rather than a dietary staple.

The Take-Home Message:
- Keep grains to a minimum. Healthy grains to choose include 100% whole grain quinoa, brown or wild rice, sprouted wheat, corn, millet, spelt, and kamut.
- Eat as many vegetables, in as many different colors, as possible.
- Try and limit fruit to 1-2 times per day. Fruit is nutritious but high in sugar. The best fruits to choose are berries, as they are lower on the glycemic scale than other fruits, and quite high in antioxidants.
- Add some form of protein to every meal, including every snack. If you eat animal products, choose organic and free-range if you can afford it. Avoid purchasing agriculture industry animal products. Other healthy proteins include tofu (non-GMO of course), nuts and nut butters, beans and hummus, yogurt (especially Greek), and fish (choose wild-caught varieties from Alaskan or Pacific waters. Avoid farm raised). Quinoa is also high in protein, for a grain.
- Cook with healthy fats, appropriate to the heat setting you're using.
- Read labels: avoid added sugar and ingredients you don't recognize. Lists should consist primarily of whole foods.

Chapter 10

BUILDING BLOCK #2: MICRONUTRIENTS

M icronutrients are the other part of the nutritional equation that your
body needs.

A *nutrient* is a catch-all term for any substance that provides the building
blocks for replenishment of an organism. It includes vitamins, minerals, essential
fatty acids, essential amino acids, and also macronutrients, such as carbs, protein,
and fats.

Vitamins and *minerals* (those nutrients normally found in a multivitamin)
are distinct from macronutrients in that they don't provide energy; rather, they
help the body carry out some of its vital functions (hence the prefix *vita-*, as
in vitality). A vitamin is a more complex molecule, while a mineral is a single
element in the periodic table. Minerals are usually combined with other things
to make them more absorbable. What it's bound to makes a difference in terms
of its bioavailability.

Once upon a time, we could get all of these nutrients straight from our diets.
Unfortunately for most of us, that's no longer true. Here's why.

Soil Requirements for Healthy Plants

Plants need essential nutrients from soil just like you need them from your food—some in large amounts, and some in trace amounts. Primary nutrients for plants include nitrogen, phosphorus and potassium. If you look at commercial fertilizer bags, the label will usually say N-P-K, representing these major nutritional requirements.

Intermediate nutrient requirements are sulfur, magnesium, and calcium.

Micronutrients include boron, copper, iron, chloride, manganese, molybdenum, zinc, cobalt, and nickel.

Too little of any one of them can affect the health of the plant, and its nutrient value to its consumers.

What Affects Nutrient Content in Soil

A few variables affect the nutrient content in the soil. One is soil texture: basically the more the soil holds on to water (moisture and stickiness), the more it will hold on to nutrients as well. Sand obviously doesn't grow much (hence the barren deserts), while clay and organic soil do.

Another important factor is soil pH. Just like our bodies have to maintain the right pH for life, so soil has to stay in the right pH range (6.0-6.5) to release both macro and micronutrients from the soil to the plants. Otherwise these nutrients will be bound up and unavailable. The right pH will also allow growth of microbe populations that help to convert the nutrients nitrogen and sulfur into usable forms for the plant. (By the way, you need plenty of microbes to help you with your digestion too!)

Fertilizer: What To Do When Soil is Suboptimal

If your soil lacks either the nutrients or the pH for growth (or both), the farmer has to fertilize. This is where the difference between commercial and organic farming comes in.

Commercial fertilizers are processed to adjust the pH rapidly and provide a walloping dose of synthetic nutrients. They are great for giving a jump-start to very depleted soil. These nutrients are mined, chemically processed, and delivered to the soil in salt form (much like our table salt, made from rock salt).

These salts release their nutrients to the soil quickly and easily when they come in contact with water.

The problem is, these fertilizers add primarily macronutrients for the plant's use, but they don't help the soil to cultivate those necessary micronutrients. (Think of it like a human subsisting entirely on fast food. You may be getting all three of the major macronutrients: carbs, protein, and fat, but you're still malnourished, and it will catch up with you eventually.) In the same way, this means that even though the plants may grow rapidly (just like you would on a fast food diet!), over time the soil gets depleted of its micronutrients. Maybe the first generation of plants grown in that soil will have all they need, but eventually those micronutrients get consumed and the soil will thus become unhealthy. This means future generations will lack those micronutrients necessary for the health of the plants, and they'll pass these deficiencies on to you.

If that weren't enough, sickly plants also tend to become targets for pests, which makes pesticides increasingly necessary (many of which are toxic to humans. As a side note on this: notice that the healthier the soil, the more easily they repel pests on their own, just like healthy humans will require far less outside assistance to prevent illness. Antibiotics, like pesticides, will work in a pinch... but they aren't dealing with the underlying issue, which is why the susceptibility exists in the first place.)

Genetically modified foods (GMO) try to get around the pest issue by adding pesticides directly to the genetic code of the plants... but among other potential problems, evidence demonstrates that GMO foods bind micronutrients such as manganese, zinc, and iron. (Not only is the soil deficient in them, but now what is there isn't available either.) This means sickly plants, sickly animals who eat the plants (since many commercial farming animals are fed from GMO corn or soy), and sickly people who eat those animals. Again, more on this in Chapter 1.

Organic Foods

Organic fertilizers are created from "natural" substances, rather than in a chemistry lab. These include things like compost, animal manure or guano, blood meal (from powdered blood), fish meal (from ground up fish), bone meal (what it sounds like), and that sort of thing. (So if you think about it… organic plants are sort of carnivorous!)

Because these nutrients are bound up in complex molecules, though, it takes time for soil organisms to decompose the organic fertilizers enough to release their key nutrients into the soil. Really depleted soil will appear to respond much faster to synthetics for this reason, but that approach doesn't aid the health of the soil and the plants in the long run. It's much better to build up the soil with compost, and then fertilize it with organic materials containing all the necessary micronutrients.

Because of this, organic foods are more nutrient dense than their commercial counterparts.[1] If you eat only organic foods (or better yet, if you live on a farm and grow your own), you may be one of the lucky few in our society who doesn't need to supplement with additional micronutrients.

Eating 100% organic is pretty expensive and not possible for most of us, though. Realistically speaking, because our food is nowhere near as nutrient dense as it used to be, most of us should be on a high quality, absorbable multivitamin to maintain health.

I look for three main things to determine whether a multivitamin is good or not. First, it should have chelated mineral forms (i.e. look at the magnesium and the calcium and etc: they should be complexed with glycinate, citrate, orotate, taurate, or another chelated form—but not oxide, carbonate, or sulfate, as these are not absorbable.) Second, dosing recommendations should specify multiple times daily. That doesn't mean you have to actually take it multiple times daily; it just means the manufacturer is aware that some of the vitamins are water-soluble, and therefore to maintain a sustained level throughout the day, you should take it more than once. And third, with the exception of whole-foods based vitamins, which are often tablets, you should choose capsules over tablets (particularly if you are older or have low stomach acid). This is because tablets are harder for your gut to break down.

Essential Fatty Acids

Almost everyone should take essential fatty acid supplements. They're called *essential* because your body can't synthesize them on its own—you have to ingest them from your diet. And unfortunately, as mentioned in the last chapter, the Standard American Diet has precious few of them. Across the population, average dietary intake of EFAs in North America tends to be around 100 mg per day, whereas healthy individuals should get around 500 mg of EFAs daily.

Probably the most important reason why everyone needs EFAs is because they are a critical component to maintaining healthy cell walls.

As mentioned in Chapter 4, historically the "brain" of the cell was considered to be its nucleus, and cell walls were considered to be the "skin." But if you remove the nucleus from a cell, it can still function just fine—it just can't reproduce (implying that the nucleus is more like the cell's reproductive organ than its brain.) But if you remove the cell's membrane, the cell dies immediately. The membrane, therefore, is even more important than the cell's nucleus!

Cell membranes are like gates, and the receptors dotted along the membrane are like gatekeepers. These receptors require a certain "password" in order to open and let a particular substance inside the cell—not just anybody gets in. But the "gate" has to be fluid enough to allow the gatekeepers to do their jobs properly, and also to let out the internal waste left over from cellular processes.

Just as we discussed for phospholipids like phosphatidylcholine and phosphatidylserine, EFAs help keep the gate fluid, letting the "good" stuff in and the "bad" stuff out. This is true for every cell in your body. Healthy cell gates will let in nutrients and oxygen (critical for life!), let in glucose for energy (limiting insulin resistance), let in neurotransmitters in brain cells (improving mood disorders), and maintain proper nerve conduction (treating neuropathy symptoms).

Letting the trash "out" is universally important too, since toxic buildup is one of the primary causes for the inflammatory diseases of Western culture, such as diabetes, heart disease, autoimmune conditions, allergies, and cancer. EFAs are also highly anti-inflammatory.

Fish oil, krill oil, or any other good EFA is comprised of EPA and DHA, which are both in the omega-3 pathway. Taking fish oil daily helps to balance out the ratio of omega-6 to omega-3.

Choosing an EFA

I prefer fish oil to flax seed oil only because the EPA content is higher in fish oil. But I still like flax seed oil, especially for vegans or vegetarians who don't eat fish.

Krill oil is a fine alternative to fish oil; it's just more expensive.

Cod liver oil has not only EFAs, but also Vitamins A and D, which is great for immune support. Depending on the brand, you might have a lower amount of EFAs than pure fish oil, but this isn't universally true.

A word of caution on fish oil: If it smells "fishy" then it's likely rancid, and rancid fish oil actually becomes a pro-oxidant, rather than an antioxidant. Don't consume capsules that have exceeded their expiration date.

When choosing an EFA supplement, look for the words "Pharmaceutical Grade" on the bottle—this means it has a much higher percentage of actual omega-3 in the capsule (compared to fillers, like fish fat).

I'd also be careful about purchasing heavily discounted fish oil. Fish can be very toxic these days, so quality matters. If you buy cheap fish oil, they probably sourced it from cheap fish—which was most likely farmed or Atlantic, both of which generally contain heavy metals.

Electrolytes

Electrolytes are another class of trace nutrients we all need for life.

The word 'electrolyte' in the context of nutrition generally refers to the largest concentration of charged particles within the human body. The biggest two are sodium (Na^+) and chloride (Cl^-), which, when combined, make up the bulk of our salt. These charged particles are critical for your physiology: all of the cells in your body do their work based on the gradient, or separation, of positive and negative charges (kind of like a battery).

This means you have to have the proper balance of electrolytes for life.

Fortunately, your body already has a pretty awesome buffer system built in to maintain these concentrations. This system kicks in when you sweat too much, drink too much reverse osmosis water (see Chapter 11), get dehydrated, or consume too much pure sodium.

The brunt of this effort to maintain your electrolyte balance falls on your kidneys. You've got to help them out, though—otherwise you'll be setting yourself up for kidney stones and osteoporosis. When dehydrated, it's important that you rehydrate not just with pure water, but also with a balance of electrolytes. This is why most sport drinks also contain electrolytes for rehydration, and why it's a good idea to use Pedialyte or a similar product when rehydrating after a bout of acute diarrhea or vomiting.

For general maintenance, it's also important to support your kidneys by taking in a good balance of electrolytes. Sodium content in processed foods is usually very high, so be careful not to consume too much. However, for those people who avoid processed foods, you may benefit from adding sea salt to your diet.

Sea Salt vs Table Salt

Historically, naturally occurring salt was the only salt available for use. This salt comes from the sea, or from other water sources (such as the Himalayas—hence the popular pink Himalayan salt). This salt contains sodium chloride and number of other trace minerals. The precise balance of minerals depends on where the salt was harvested from. Usually they include a combination of silicon and phosphorus (both necessary for calcium uptake into bones), vanadium (which helps with blood sugar control), magnesium (a very common deficiency), calcium, and potassium.

By contrast, most of the salt on American tables is more highly processed. It begins as rock salt, and is heated in a kiln to 1200 degrees F to remove impurities, changing its chemical structure to sodium chloride (NaCl—processed salt is about 98% this). Then they add anti-caking agents (such as toxic ferrocyanide and aluminosilicate), and in places where there isn't fluorine added to the water, they'll add fluoride to the salt, plus a little potassium iodide (added because we're not getting enough iodine in our diets). In other words, table salt lacks the trace minerals of sea salt, and contains chemical additives your body doesn't need (although for those with low iodine levels, iodized sea salt is not a bad idea).

As a general rule, you should avoid any highly processed substance that masquerades as food. In this case, though, by choosing sea salt, you'll also get a good source of other electrolytes and minerals, which will assist your kidneys in maintaining optimum health.

Antioxidants

We know that oxidative stress is a mediating factor in heart disease, diabetes, cancer, Alzheimer's disease, and chronic inflammatory diseases, and it is postulated to be a major contributor to cellular aging as well. Antioxidants neutralize the free radicals (unpaired electrons) that cause oxidative stress. Many nutrients are considered to be antioxidants, but most important are those found throughout the body (called "endogenous"), and those that are capable of regenerating other antioxidants. To protect yourself against the oxidative damage rampant in our modern world, choose a complex that contains NAC (N-Acetyl Cysteine), ALA (Alpha Lipoic Acid), and/or CoQ10. There are also specific antioxidants which may be important for a given condition, but it's best to check with your naturopathic doctor which ones are right for you.

Probiotics

Medical professionals are realizing more and more that your gut is the gateway not just to pathogenic illnesses, but also to noninfectious gut disorders like allergies and autoimmunity. It's also the key to protecting against these ailments (that's why you're reading this book!)

Although it may seem unnatural to supplement with microorganisms, people once consumed a much higher volume of fermented foods (and therefore of probiotics) than they do today. Look for a probiotic with 20 billion organisms at about a 50/50 ratio of Lactobacillus and Bifidobacterium, as these are the organisms that make up the majority of the Western culture gut flora.

Individual Micronutrient Deficiencies

These basic supplement recommendations presuppose an otherwise healthy body. In some cases, though, people need more of a particular nutrient to correct a problem. In general, do not supplement an individual vitamin or mineral without testing or the advice of a nutritionist or naturopathic physician, because overdose or imbalance is possible for some of them, and also because some of these symptoms may be indicative of an underlying condition that you might mask with supplementation.

That said, one nutrient stands out as a frequent deficiency in my patients with gut health issues.

Magnesium Deficiency

Magnesium is a cofactor for about 300 reactions in your body (meaning it's required for the reaction to proceed). These reactions include making, transporting, and using energy, making DNA and proteins, controlling nerve signals, relaxing muscles, and responding adequately to stress.

Reasons You Might Be Low

You might not be eating enough of the foods that contain magnesium. Magnesium is found in whole grains, nuts, beans, green leafy veggies, fish, and (clean) meat.

Even if you're consuming plenty of these foods, a bunch of pharmaceuticals also block the absorption of magnesium or increase its excretion, including laxatives, diuretics, proton pump inhibitors (like Nexium), antibiotics, colchicine, and corticosteroids (like prednisone).

You can also deplete magnesium by consuming too much alcohol or too many phosphates (from soda usually).

If you have a hard time absorbing nutrients in general (a malabsorption syndrome, such as Crohn's, celiac sprue, or enteritis), then you are likely to be deficient in magnesium also.

You might be deficient if you have Type 2 Diabetes, especially if it isn't well controlled, because high blood sugar leads to increased urination, and like all electrolytes, magnesium reabsorption happens in the kidneys.

How You Know If You're Low

The test for magnesium in your bloodstream (serum magnesium) isn't reliable, because most magnesium stays inside your cells and your bones. Red blood cell (RBC) magnesium is a better test, therefore, because that's testing the magnesium concentration inside the red blood cells.

However, often clinical signs and symptoms, combined with knowledge of one of the five causes listed above is the best way to determine deficiency. Low magnesium can lead to problems with memory and concentration, depression and apathy, emotional lability (you get upset easily), irritability, nervousness, and anxiety, insomnia, constipation, migraines, PMS and cramping, fibromyalgia and muscle pain, fatigue, and ADHD.

Micronutrients Matter

Your body requires both micronutrients and macronutrients. You can't give it calories without vitamins and minerals, because the body will still tell you it wants more. It thinks you're starving it if you aren't taking in adequate micronutrients, even if you're gorging yourself on fast food every day.

The Take-Home Message:

- If organic food is available and affordable, buy it. When organic isn't available or affordable, at least go for whole foods.
- Get on a good, absorbable multivitamin.
- Start taking a pharmaceutical grade fish oil or other essential fatty acid.
- Get yourself on a probiotic.
- Consider testing for other nutrient deficiencies and supplementing appropriately.

Chapter 11

BUILDING BLOCK #3: WATER, FRESH AIR, AND SUNLIGHT

Picture a dim, musty room, with the window all boarded up and the counters and walls covered with dirt and grime. Would you be surprised if the place was infested with pests or disease?

Instinctively we just know places like that are unhealthy. If you wanted to clean up a dank space, would your first instinct be bleach and antiseptic spray? Or would you instead throw open the windows, let in some fresh air and sunlight, and hose the place down?

Our bodies are the same way. Pests and infections tend to thrive in unhealthy environments, but with some fresh air, sunlight, and plenty of clean water to flush us out, our bodies become far less hospitable to disease.

Breathe Deeply

To start, let's not even go so far as to talk about *fresh* air... right now let's just talk about *air*, period. Americans tend to be a pretty stressed out bunch, and when we get stressed, we often unconsciously quit breathing. Even if this happens only for a few seconds at a time, the effects may be cumulative.

What Happens When You Hold Your Breath

There are a few primary routes for toxin elimination. These include the urinary system, the liver, the bowels, the sweat, and the breath. We breathe in oxygen and breathe out carbon dioxide. But when we hold our breath, this delicate balance gets disrupted. Carbon dioxide accumulates in our bodies, which acts as an acid in the bloodstream. A complicated buffer system involving the kidneys has to kick in to buffer this process and keep us from becoming too acidic (the same buffer system that keeps our electrolytes in check). Without this buffering process, we would quickly go into respiratory distress, which can be very serious. Symptoms of respiratory distress include confusion, fatigue, lethargy, shortness of breath, and sleepiness.

(Sound familiar–albeit in milder form?)

What Contributes to Insufficient Breathing?

This can be as simple as the way you are sitting as you stare at your computer (like I am doing right now—I just sat up straighter as I typed this!) Proper breathing comes from your belly as your diaphragm lowers, and not from your chest. Hunching over requires you to chest-breathe, which gives you less than adequate respiration.

Another cause, of course, is stress. The autonomic "fight or flight" response leads to short, shallow breathing; "rest and digest" promotes deep belly breathing. Stress can be caused by something as simple as overwhelming amounts of email (which led to the term, "email apnea." No, I didn't make that up.) A constant sense of urgency interrupts your body's oxygen/carbon dioxide balance.

The Solution

One of the most well-known and least utilized tricks for coping with anxiety is deep breathing. Sit up straight; put your hand on your belly to remind yourself to breathe from there and not from your chest. Close your eyes, and count as you inhale (and your belly expands) to 8 or 10 or whatever number feels right to you, but don't rush it. Then exhale just as completely, and for the same count. Do this a few times and you will feel yourself become much more relaxed.

It's a good idea to practice this technique throughout the day. You may not have to close your eyes and count, as long as you breathe consciously and on purpose. Or, join a gentle stretching or exercise class such as yoga or Tai Chi, where breathing is a central component of the movement. I know I feel a sort of euphoria after these classes, and while some of it is undoubtedly due to the movement itself, much of it is likely due to a greater supply of oxygen to the brain than I typically get!

Drink Water

Sometimes we forget about water as a key component to our health. It's easy to forget, because it's so readily available. But water plays a vital role in almost every system of our bodies. This makes sense, because about 80% of our bodies are comprised of water. Water comprises about 70% of lean muscle, about 80% of our blood, and roughly 85% of our brain volume.

The Effect of Water on Blood

When I have a patient with low blood pressure, my first question is, "How much water have you been drinking?" Low fluid intake equals low blood volume. Low blood volume can equal low blood pressure, and thus lower blood flow to your organs (decreasing the supply of oxygen and nutrients and elimination of waste from those tissues). Patients with low blood pressure and blood volume frequently say they experience the room going dark for a few seconds when they stand up too quickly—it takes a bit longer for the blood to get to their brains from the sudden shift in position. (This is also often an indication of adrenal fatigue—see Chapter 5).

The Effect of Water on Toxins

One of the main purposes of water is to assist in the elimination of waste. This happens not just in the bloodstream (because more blood means flushing out those tissues faster), but it also helps to flush out the organs of elimination, such as the liver, kidneys, and bowels. (Think of it this way. When something on the *outside* of your body is dirty, what do you use to flush it out?)

Low water intake leads to low urine output and constipation—which means toxins are not getting out of your body effectively. Toxin accumulation can lead to all kinds of symptoms, depending on what the toxin is and where your susceptibilities lie (see Chapters 1-5).

The Symptoms of Dehydration

Low water intake can lead to dehydration, of course, and acute dehydration can be severe and even fatal. Symptoms of dehydration can include a fast heart rate to compensate for low blood volume and blood pressure, fast breathing to compensate for lower oxygen delivery to the tissues, dry mouth, and eventually loss of consciousness. Symptoms of chronic dehydration include constipation (this is one of the first things to consider if you are constipated), headache (remember that 85% of our brains are water), and muscle cramping, since dehydration leads to an imbalance in some of the key electrolytes such as magnesium, potassium, chloride, calcium, and sodium. Electrolyte imbalances are usually responsible for muscle cramps.

Different Types of Water

All water sources are not created equal. Here's the breakdown of different sources.

Tap Water

We've all heard how contaminated our tap water is. If you're curious to know what's in the water supply near you, go to the Environmental Working Group's website (at http://www.ewg.org/tap-water/whats-in-yourwater.php) and type in your zip code. In my area, the contaminants that exceed health guidelines include arsenic, lead, radioactive alpha particles, and four disinfectant byproducts formed as a result of chlorine or other disinfectants. Quite a few other contaminants were detected below the health limit levels.

So, tap water isn't the best option in all areas of the country. But even tap water is better than being dehydrated.

Bottled Water

Although bottled water seems to be cleaner than tap water, according to the NRDC, some 25% of bottled water also contains too-high levels of at least one contaminant.

But more importantly, most single-use bottled water is sold in flimsy plastic bottles, a common source of phthalates. Phthalates are not only estrogenic, they have been found to increase programmed cell death (particularly in testicular cells). Overall, phthalates are linked to breast cancer, birth defects, low sperm count, obesity, diabetes, and thyroid problems. (More on this in Chapter 2.) The stiffer the plastic, however, the less of an issue phthalates become.

Delivery-based water services are a better option than tap water for many of us who live in areas where the tap water is less than ideal. However, patients can have varying sensitivities to the phthalates, as shown in Leanne's case below.

Case Study:

I hadn't seen Leanne for over a year when she came back to my clinic. She returned because suddenly her period became about three times heavier than usual. "I'm bleeding like a stuck pig!" was her somewhat colorful description.

It seemed very strange that a normal cycle would alter so abruptly in a single month, so I questioned her about what had changed. I asked if she'd started using plastics for her food or her water bottle. Her eyes grew wide. "Actually, yes!" She told me the glass water bottle she normally used had broken about a month earlier, and she'd intended to replace it but hadn't gotten around to it. Instead, she'd been using a plastic one she carried in her purse, refilling it multiple times daily.

"Bingo," I said. It was June in Tucson, AZ, so the phthalate content in the water was likely even worse than usual, as the heat encourages phthalates to leech into the water.

I suggested she buy a glass or stainless steel water bottle ASAP, and also prescribed a detox protocol including sauna, hydrotherapy, castor oil packs, and enemas. For good measure, I put her on Chaste Tree to help normalize her cycle.

Sure enough, Leanne's next period returned to normal.

Filtered Water

You can buy pitchers, bottles, or faucet attachments to filter your tap water. These will remove chlorine (and therefore chlorine byproducts), and positively charged ions such as copper, cadmium, mercury, and lead.

This can be an easy and cheap solution for many people.

Reverse Osmosis Water

Reverse Osmosis water is the best way to ensure that the highest percentage of all contaminants are removed from your water.

The main concern I have with reverse osmosis water is that it also removes necessary minerals like electrolytes, which we most definitely need. If this is your only source of electrolytes, you might end up with some imbalances. I always suggest these patients add at least one electrolyte replacement packet to their water per day.

Kangen Water

This very expensive filtration system ionizes water, rendering your drinking water alkaline to the tune of 8.5-9.5 pH. The idea is that it will help your body to become more alkaline—implying that regular water might have the opposite effect, taxing the body's pH buffering system in order to neutralize it.

However, because water has a pH right around 7 (which is neutral, like most of the fluids in your body), it should not activate the buffering systems at all, and therefore should not cause a problem. So as far as I can tell, Kangen water systems are unnecessary.

Sunlight

Most of us experience a sense of enjoyment from being outdoors when the weather is comfortable. We feel better outside—there's something refreshing about being out in nature. There are good medical reasons for this.

Vitamin D (some of which is ingested in the diet, but 90-95% of which comes from sunlight) has been the darling of the nutritional world for years now.

The Benefits of Vitamin D

- *It's Anti-Cancer.* Over 2000 studies link deficiency of Vitamin D to cancer, and one study[1] suggests that keeping Vitamin D levels at just 40 ng/mL lowers overall cancer risk by about 77%. Another study[2] suggests that a serum level of 55–60 ng/mL may reduce the breast cancer rate by *half* in temperate climates.
- *It lowers the risk of diabetes.* Low vitamin D is linked more closely to diabetes than is obesity.[3]
- *It lowers the risk of Multiple Sclerosis (MS).* MS occurs a lot less often in sunny places than in dark and gloomy ones.[4]
- *It reduces PMS and period cramping.* Apparently Vitamin D is anti-inflammatory, too—and inflammation is responsible for the cramping of PMS.[5] This suggests any inflammatory condition can improve with a healthy dose of Vitamin D.

Why the Chronic Vitamin D Deficiency?

I like to see my patients maintain Vitamin D levels of at least 40 ng/mL. But almost every patient I test is low in Vitamin D unless they're supplementing with it. This is true even though I live in Arizona, where it's sunny nearly all the time. So what gives?

Physiology 101 on Vitamin D

When we're exposed to UVB rays from the sun, the sebum on our skin creates 7-dehydrocholesterol. This process takes about 48 hours. Then 7-dehydrocholesterol enters the bloodstream, where it follows a complex series of chemical pathways performed by the liver and kidneys. The 7-dehydrocholesterol finally becomes calcitriol, whose main job is to increase calcium absorption from food.

The most obvious issue here is the length of time this takes. Most of us shower daily, which means we're washing off the sebum before it has a chance to turn our sun exposure into the vitamin D precursor necessary to begin this process.

Even the amount that does enter the bloodstream has a few hurdles to overcome. As we've discovered throughout this book, all of the nutrients in your body influence one another, either directly or indirectly. Tamper with one and you can cause repercussions elsewhere. Also, keep in mind that your body is a living system, always seeking balance. So if, for example, your tissue levels of calcium are higher than they should be, your body may shut down calcitriol production in the kidneys to try to achieve that balance.

Why Tissue Burden of Calcium Might be High

A study came out a few years ago that suggested calcium supplementation could increase the risk of heart attacks.[6] The concern here is that atherosclerotic plaques contain calcium deposits, and it was hypothesized that taking calcium in supplement form could contribute to plaque formation. (The study measured non-absorbable forms of calcium, such as calcium oxide or sulfate, and not the absorbable forms found in appropriate ratios with other nutrients necessary for bone deposition. But the concern that too much calcium can precipitate out onto body tissues is real.[7])

Researchers feared that we might have too much calcium in our tissues and not enough in our bones due to our highly acidic diets in the US. As mentioned above, the buffering system gets activated in response to substances that have an acidifying effect on the body, in order to maintain the optimum blood pH. Foods with an acidic effect on the body buffering systems include beef, ice cream, canned fruits, peanuts, bacon, tuna, corn, sugar, vinegar, corn syrup, cereals, mustard, mayo, corn tortillas, milk, sardines, soft drinks, artificial sweeteners, and ketchup.

Foods with an alkalinizing effect include alfalfa, celery, barley grass, peppers, beet greens, broccoli, cabbage, mustard greens, chard greens, collard greens, chlorella, onions, cucumber, spinach, spirulina, garlic, green beans, dandelions, lettuce, kohlrabi, kale, pumpkin, wheat grass, sprouts, watercress, and wild greens.

So basically our calcium is in the wrong place: it's in our tissues rather than our bones, because our bodies have pulled it from our bones in order to counteract our highly acidic diets. This may dial down our vitamin D production, even in the presence of adequate sunlight: because our bodies are saying, "Stop with the calcium already!"

The point here is not to stop taking your calcium supplements, provided you are taking a chelated form (glycinate, citrate, orotate, etc), and it is complexed with other components required for bone deposition. The point, rather, is that one potential cause of low Vitamin D might be high calcium in the bloodstream, secondary to an acidic diet. Shift your dietary intake from the acidic foods listed above to those with an alkalinizing effect to help lower tissue burden of calcium, and Vitamin D may rebound.

Vitamin K and Calcium
Vitamin K is another fat-soluble vitamin like Vitamin D, and its job is to allow the body to take calcium and use it in the clotting cascade. Vitamin K also produces a protein called osteocalcin, which puts calcium into the bones.

You get vitamin K1 from super-healthy veggies (broccoli, turnips, cabbage, cauliflower, and spinach), and then it gets converted to the active Vitamin K2 by the good bacteria in your gut. But alas, most of us aren't eating those veggies, and we also don't have nearly as much good bacteria in our guts as we ought to (and often we have a lot of bad bacteria instead). Result: too little vitamin K —> too much calcium in the tissues (rather than in the bones and clotting cascade, where it's supposed to be.)

Again, the message here: eat plenty of cruciferous veggies, and take your probiotics to have an adequate balance of Vitamin K1 and K2 in order to keep calcium where it needs to be. I'd also recommend that any calcium supplement you take include Vitamin K2 as well.

How Magnesium is connected to Calcium and Vitamin D
Like Vitamin D, magnesium also helps to regulate calcium levels, because magnesium and calcium have opposite effects. (Calcium and magnesium should remain in about a 2:1 ratio.) But if you don't have enough magnesium (and it's a common deficiency, as addressed in Chapter 10), your tissue levels of calcium go up, too.

Magnesium is also used in the metabolism of Vitamin D, so too little magnesium can lead to low Vitamin D that way, also. Make sure your absorbable calcium supplement also includes magnesium.

To Raise Vitamin D Levels:
- Get your levels tested, and if you bathe daily, you will likely need to supplement at least a maintenance dose (about 2000 IU daily).
- If you want to increase your vitamin D levels through sun exposure, your best bet is to 1) wash only those parts of you that require special attention with soap and just rinse off elsewhere; 2) bare as much skin as the weather comfortably allows, and 3) stay in the sun (careful of overheating, of course) until you start to turn just slightly pink. (Any longer and you will burn, which can set you up for skin cancers.)
- If you are at risk for osteopenia, take an absorbable form of calcium (NOT oxide, sulfate, or carbonate) complexed at least with adequate magnesium and Vitamin K2.
- Shift your dietary intake towards alkaline foods and away from acidic foods.

While it is important to get enough sunlight for adequate Vitamin D production, I hope you're getting the message that *all healthy habits work together in concert.* In order for sunlight's production of Vitamin D to be as effective as possible, you also need to consume a healthy diet and balance your micronutrients.

The sun does more than just boost your Vitamin D levels, though.

Some forms of depression are directly linked to low Vitamin D (Seasonal Affective Disorder). Even aside from that, **sun exposure boosts serotonin,** the "feel-good" neurotransmitter.

One study[6] shows that exposure to UVB rays increases production if nitric oxide, which causes blood vessels to dilate, thus **lowering blood pressure.**

Exposure to sunlight early in the morning helps your body to produce melatonin earlier, making it **easier to sleep** at the end of the day.[7]

The Take-Home Message:

- **Drink clean, filtered water.** Half your body weight in ounces is a good rule of thumb (so if you weigh 140 lbs, you should be drinking 70 oz of water daily), but you should increase that number if you are out in the summer heat or exercising (which you should be—see chapter 13!) This is one of the simplest and most important things you can do for your health.
- **Breathe deeply!** This helps your body to remain alkaline.
- **Eat whole foods,** to minimize acidity in your body.
- **Spend 5-15 minutes a day in the sun, without sunblock, three times per week in the spring and summertime (and an hour in the winter).** Longer sun exposures aren't necessary—there are diminishing returns after that point, increasing the risk of aging from the sun and skin cancers, but not improving Vitamin D Status. This will help to boost your Vitamin D levels, boost your serotonin, boost your nitric oxide, lower inflammation, and generally make you healthier!

Chapter 12

Building Block #4: Sleep

We all feel better when we get enough sleep.

But sometimes it's hard to prioritize sleep when there are other things you'd rather accomplish, or things that have to get done. According to the CDC, some 40% of Americans are chronically sleep deprived[1]—defined as unintentionally nodding off at least once during the previous month!

Getting adequate sleep for your age and body is one of the absolute foundational health requirements. Here are some of the things plenty of sleep does for you (and that lack of sleep can deprive you of):

Sleep improves your memory. Remember those commercials years ago when Candace Bergen that every time you learn something, it makes a new "wrinkle in your brain?" This reorganization of the brain's structure when both learning something new and consolidating that memory is known as neuroplasticity, and sleep is a necessary part of this process. You may even practice new skills in your dreams, which strengthens that new neural pathway and makes those same skills easier to perform in your waking hours.

On the other hand, why does sleep deprivation cause memory problems? One possible (chilling) explanation is that sleep gives your brain time to "clean up" toxic proteins that can accumulate throughout waking hours, including beta amyloid and tau—the proteins linked with Alzheimer's Disease. In one study[2], mice who were only allowed to sleep four hours per night were not only impaired in their ability to recall and learn new tasks, they were found to have an increased level of tau proteins in their brains.

Sleep helps you live longer. The reasons for this are not entirely clear, but it may have to do with the hormone melatonin (the "sleep hormone"), which is a powerful antioxidant, among other things. Insufficient sleep is also correlated with higher levels of inflammation, and therefore higher incidence of hypertension and cardiovascular disease. Even in the short term, sleep deprivation is correlated with dramatically reduced immune function.

Sleep affects your blood sugar. Poor blood sugar control and high cortisol can both also set you up for overgrowth of yeast, and leaky gut syndrome. Consistently getting less than 6 hours of sleep per night is also correlated with a higher BMI (basal metabolic index)—which means it's harder to lose weight if you're not sleeping enough. This is because during sleep, your body secretes hormones that regulate appetite and blood sugar. Insufficient sleep leads to an increase in the hunger hormone ghrelin, a decrease in the satiety hormone leptin, and an increase in cortisol, the stress hormone, which (among other things) increases your blood sugar. Lack of sleep can therefore lead to obesity, poor blood sugar control, and even diabetes. (Conversely, 8 hours of sleep per night is correlated with a lower BMI.)

Sleep improves performance, at whatever you do—be it athletics, school, work, or creative endeavors. This probably has to do with that feeling of drowsiness, which is at least partly due to the accumulation of adenosine, a by-product of neuronal activity which builds up during waking hours and leads to the feeling of being tired. (Caffeine works by blocking the adenosine receptors, as well as indirectly pumping out more adrenaline to keep you going even when your adenosine levels are high.)

Sleep prevents accidents. Probably also in part due to the accumulation of adenosine in the brain, driving under the effects of drowsiness is responsible for 20 percent of all car accidents, causing 8000 deaths yearly in the US. In some cases it is considered even more dangerous than driving under the influence of alcohol.

Sleep helps to restore and rejuvenate tissues. Many physiologic activities are reduced during sleep, but some are increased. One such activity is the release of growth hormone (GH), which helps to repair muscles and tissues from the normal wear-and-tear of everyday living. (For this reason, conditions like fibromyalgia, or chronic muscle pain, are correlated with insufficient sleep—and therefore insufficient GH to repair muscles.)

Adequate Sleep

How much sleep do you need to reap these benefits and avoid these pitfalls? According to the National Sleep Foundation, there's a range based on your age and your genetics.

- *Newborns (0-3 mo):* 14-17 hours is average, but the range can go anywhere from 11-19 hours
- *Infants (4-11 mo):* 12-15 hours average, 10-18 hours may apply
- *Toddlers (1-2 years):* 11-14 hours average, 9-16 hours may apply
- *Preschool (3-5 years):* 10-13 hours average, 8-14 hours may apply
- *School age (6-13 years):* 9-11 hours average, 7-12 hours may apply
- *Teenagers (14-17 years):* 8-10 hours average, 7-11 hours may apply
- *Young adults (18-25 years):* 7-9 hours average, 6-11 hours may apply
- *Adults (26-64 years):* 7-9 hours average, 6-10 hours may apply
- *Older adults (65 and over):* 7-8 hours average, 5-9 hours may apply.

My advice on finding the right number of hours for you: on a day when you're not already sleep-deprived, turn off your alarm and see how many hours you sleep. That's probably your ideal number. Our world doesn't really make it easy to sleep nine hours per night as an adult, so I recommend finding an average number at which you can function well and sticking to it. For example: if nine is ideal for you, but you can function well on eight but no less, then make eight your minimum. Every now and then things come up and you won't even be able to achieve eight, though. If that happens, do a little math for the subsequent nights that week. If one night you only get five hours, then you're at a deficit of three—so you need to get those three in over the rest of the week, plus your eight for each of the subsequent nights. That means you can either sleep eleven the very next night, or ten the next night and nine the night after, or nine the three following nights.

That should be enough to help you average out, and prevent the deficits from stacking up.

Good Sleep Hygiene

If you struggle with insomnia, before trying supplements and medications, make sure you've done all the basic stuff first.

Try to go to bed at the same time every night and wake up at the same time every morning, even if you're not tired at night and/or got very little sleep by morning. It is best to wake with the sun in order to reset your biological clock, spend a few minutes in the early morning sunlight, and then go to bed early enough that this will give you as many hours as you need to feel your best. Night shift workers need to maintain as regular a schedule as possible to give their internal clocks a chance to adjust, and many of them may adjust faster if they sleep before going to work instead of after, or nap beforehand as well as after, in order to mimic the normal shift schedule of going to work shortly after rising.

If you cannot fall asleep, get up and do something else. The anxiety of trying to fall asleep can actually exacerbate the problem.

The last hour (or at least half an hour) before you go to bed, do something very calming— read a book, listen to music, pray, or meditate in bed until you start to nod off. Try not to watch TV or stare at a computer screen right before bed, as the blue light decreases melatonin production. Do not take any stimulants or engage in stimulating activities before bed.

Have a cup of tea (chamomile is my favorite) while you do this, and try to slow down your breathing. Alternatively, you can try having a cup of warm (organic!) milk right before bed, with a pinch of nutmeg or turmeric. If you are sensitive to dairy, try warm soy milk (non-GMO!), almond milk, coconut milk, flax milk, rice milk, or hemp milk instead.

Consume little or no alcohol before bedtime. Alcohol may help you fall into a light sleep, but it maintains only lighter stages and prevents REM and deeper stages of sleep. This means you can be awakened more easily. This is why drinking alcohol before bed is associated with waking in the middle of the night.

Give up smoking. Like those who have alcohol right before bed, smokers tend to sleep very lightly, and wake after 3-4 hours of sleep due to the nicotine withdrawal.

Avoid caffeine after 2 pm. In theory, the half life of caffeine in the bloodstream is four hours, but this actually depends on the individual's metabolic rate. Some people process caffeine faster and some slower. It's best to err on the side of caution.

Are you taking supplements right before bed? Make sure there are no stimulants in them. This includes B vitamins and even vitamin C for some patients.

Get enough exercise: 20-30 minutes per day.

Keep your room cool—you lose your ability to regulate body temperature during REM, so abnormally hot or cold temperatures in the environment can disrupt this stage of sleep.

Some people have difficulty sleeping due to an overabundance of thoughts. If you find that you cannot help but continue to problem-solve, **get out of bed and write your thoughts down on a piece of paper** until you can think of no more. I'd also highly recommend counting backwards from 1000. It's hard to maintain a logical train of thought at the same time!

Resist getting up to go to the bathroom if you wake up in the middle of the night. Bladders are always full at night, but it shouldn't wake you up, nor should it keep you awake. Usually when you feel like you have to go, if you ignore it, you will drift off to sleep anyway.

Put the bedroom clock out of arm's reach and facing away from you so you can't see it. This may help for two reasons: one, it decreases the anxiety associated with the hour, and two, some people are especially light sensitive and need total darkness to sleep their best. The light can actually disrupt the production of melatonin.

Have a light snack before bedtime so you're not hungry. Hunger is a cause of insomnia in many animals, including humans. This is especially true if you find yourself consistently waking between 2-3 am. It's best to make this something high in healthy fat or protein to help stabilize blood sugar.

Try not to nap much after 2 pm if possible.

The Right Kind of Sleep

Although we hear about REM sleep more often than other stages because it is associated with dreams, there are actually five stages of sleep: 1, 2, 3, 4, and REM, which occurs between stages 1 and 2. Stages 3 and 4 are the deepest stages. Without adequate sleep in stages 3 and 4, people wake feeling groggy and "hung over"—even if you hit your ideal number of hours. My favorite natural remedy to get people into stages 3 and 4 (assuming they're already not drinking alcohol before bedtime—if so, cut that out) is the amino acid and neurotransmitter glycine[3]. I usually recommend a powdered version, since it's easier to take a lot of it; 3 grams an hour before bedtime works well to help propel patients into REM and stage 3-4 sleep.

More stubborn cases of insomnia may require individual neurotransmitter testing and supplementation based on lab results, hormone balancing, and/or individualized homeopathic prescriptions. For patients who have never been on long-term sleep medications, this is usually sufficient. For patients who already have a dependency on sleep meds such as Ambien, Lorazepam, Trazodone, Lunesta, etc—it's possible to get off, but it's usually a process of finding the right taper schedule (or even switching to less addictive meds and then tapering off of those) combined with the right additional supplements to help reset your body's natural sleep cycle. Long-term sleep medication users typically require a long drawn out taper process, so be patient.

The Take-Home Message:

- Find your ideal number of hours of sleep per night, based upon the hours you sleep without an alarm when you are not already at a sleep deficit. Make this your average number of hours per night—which means, if you get less than that number one night, pay the debt back over the next night or few nights.

- Go to bed at the same time every night, and wake up around the same time every day.
- Have a wind-down routine. Turn off screens and do something calming, with low lighting, for at least 30 minutes before your bedtime.
- Start exercising if you're not already!
- If you need more help on getting adequate sleep, consider seeing a functional medicine practitioner or a naturopathic doctor to help you dig in to the root cause—particularly checking your cortisol levels at night and your neurotransmitters.

Chapter 13

BUILDING BLOCK #5: EXERCISE

Bowel irregularity is unfortunately super common in industrialized countries. Much of this has to do with the Standard American Diet, which is high in processed foods and sugar, and low in fiber. However, the more exercise you get, the more toned your core muscles become and the better your bowels tend to move. This helps prevent slow bowel transit, dysbiosis, and digestive inflammation that can lead to deeper nutrient malabsorption issues. It also helps you to sleep better, which reduces your stress, balances your cortisol, and also improves gut function!

It can be hard to start a new routine. But if you can find a buddy to help keep you accountable and motivated for those first 21 days (which is about the length of time necessary to create a new habit), regular exercise is probably the very best thing you can do to improve not only your gut, but also your mood, and your joint health. It will also help you to lose weight, lower blood pressure and cholesterol levels, and of course, look and feel better!

If you hate exercise, it may be because you're not used to it. Everyone can find some form of physical activity that they enjoy if they're determined. Do you love the beauty of nature? Go for a walk or a hike in the evening when it gets cool, or in the morning as the sun rises. Do you enjoy calming stretches? Sign up for a yoga class. Do you enjoy fluid movement? Consider taking up dancing! Really, there's something for everyone. Start slow, but make it a habit. That's the key.

Okay, on to the specifics. The three components of fitness are aerobic (cardiovascular), strength, and flexibility. Most forms of physical activity will provide some benefits in all three areas.

Aerobic

Aerobic exercises are those that involve repetitive motions of large muscle groups. These include walking, jogging, swimming, bicycling, Elliptical machines, aerobics classes, dancing, hiking, and rowing machines. Of course, if you haven't exercised in awhile, make sure you start with gentle walking and work your way up, or see your doctor to determine whether a particular exercise program is right for you. Assuming you're already active, though, here's how to do aerobic exercise correctly.

Before you start, calculate your target heart rate zone to make sure you achieve the benefits of aerobic exercise. Maximum heart rate can be calculated as approximately 220 beats per minute, minus your age. Multiply this number by 0.6 in order to yield 60% of your maximum heart rate, or by 0.8 in order to yield 80% of your maximum heart rate. **The target heart rate range for maximum benefits is 60-80%.** As long as you keep your heart beating at a rate of between 60-80% for at least 20 minutes, the benefits of aerobic exercise will be attained.

The easiest way to determine your heart rate is to count the number of beats in 15 seconds (measured at the wrist or in the neck) and multiply by four to give beats per minute. For example, if you count 22 beats in 15 seconds, your heart rate would be 88 (22 x 4) bpm. You can perform this calculation while exercising to determine whether you are in the desired range, or you can use exercise monitors specifically designed to measure this for you.

The intensity of exercise required to reach your target heart rate will vary according to your level of fitness when you begin your exercise program. If you have not exercised in some time, it won't take a lot of work to reach your target heart rate.

Any intense exercise should incorporate a warm up and cool down period. A warm up can be simply beginning your exercise at low intensity and gradually increasing to your desired intensity over five minutes. This prepares your body for aerobic exercise and prevents injuries.

Strength

Begin a strength training program that works all of the major muscle groups of the upper and lower body. Below is a list of exercises that fall into these categories. Ask the trainers at your gym to identify these machines for you if you are unfamiliar with them.

- *Upper body exercises* include bicep curls, tricep extensions, lat pull downs, seated rows, chest press/fly, shoulder press, and upright rows. You can also perform exercises for most upper body muscles using free weights.
- *Lower body exercises* include the leg press, squats, or lunges; leg curls, calf raises, and abdominal crunches.

A repetition is the number of times you repeat a particular exercise. Each time you complete this number of repetitions, it's called a set. If your goal is to lose weight or create lean muscle, lower weight and higher repetitions is recommended, while higher weight and fewer repetitions are preferred to bulk up. As a rule of thumb, most trainers recommend three sets of each exercise, with 8 to 12 repetitions.

Repetitions should be slow—lift to a count of 2 and hold at the top of the contraction for about 1 second. Lower to the count of 4. Going faster while lifting or lowering the resistance uses momentum, not muscle, which both increases the chance of injury and decreases effectiveness of the exercise.

Rest your muscles in between sets. 60-90 seconds is recommended for muscle recovery. Alternatively, in order to save time, I use my "rest" period to perform another exercise using a different muscle group (called a superset). Usually I choose the muscle group that does the opposite of the one I just worked (or the antagonistic muscle group)—for instance, I will superset bicep curls with tricep extensions.

Work each muscle group until you can't lift the weight any more without a rest. Trainers call this working the muscle to fatigue. This will ensure that you get the maximum benefits from your exercise.

Perform strength training on a given muscle group only every other day. It takes two days for your muscles to heal from microtears incurred during strength training. Many trainers recommend strength training only three days per week. Alternatively, I do some strength training daily but alternate between back/chest, upper and lower body workouts.

Increase your resistance as you gain strength. If you stop increasing resistance, your gains will plateau. This is fine, however, if you've achieved your desired level of fitness.

Stretching

Most of us think of stretching as something you do for maybe 15 seconds before you work out, to prevent muscle injury. But there's a lot more to it than that.

So many of my patients complain of neck and back pain, which nearly always starts with tight muscles. Muscles can become tight due to posture problems, overuse, repetitive movements that strain one part of the body and cause compensation elsewhere, and (often) stress—which causes us to hunch up or hunch over, as our bodies unconsciously bear our burdens for us.

Much of this could be prevented with regular stretching!

Stretching will increase blood flow. Some cultures think of blood as the "life force" of a creature, and for good reason: blood brings oxygen and nutrients to cells, and eliminates metabolic waste. So many great naturopathic therapies (also including hydrotherapy and massage) boil down to this: *increased circulation = increased vitality.* This goes for all forms of exercise too.

Stretching leads to greater flexibility. Think of it this way: if you drop a glass bottle on the ground, it shatters, because (among other things) glass has no "give". It can't absorb the impact. Conversely, if you drop a rubber ball on the ground, it bounces, because rubber can absorb the impact. You want your muscles to be more like rubber than like glass. Flexibility = "give."

Stretching increases your range of motion. The more range of motion you have, the better your balance becomes. Better balance will not only make you more graceful, but it will also prevent injury from falls.

Stretching leads to greater strength gains. Stretching may actually improve muscular performance and endurance, much the way lifting weights does.

Stretching is great for stress reduction. It forces you to slow down and breathe deeply, for one thing. It also decreases some of the secondary signs of stress, such as shoulder and neck tightness. But, as a side benefit to increased blood flow, stretching also releases the same endorphins you get from other forms of exercise—which is why a yoga class can leave you feeling euphoric!

Tips for Stretching Right

Make sure you warm up first. Contrary to popular opinion, stretching itself is not a warm-up. A "warm up" is an activity that increases blood flow to the muscles. Stretching a muscle that doesn't yet have that extra influx of oxygen from increased blood flow can actually cause injury. It's a better idea to stretch your muscles after your workout, instead of before… or to at least "warm up" with some light cardio before stretching.

Stretch for symmetry. Especially if one side of your body tends to have issues more than the other (which is most of us,) stretching can help to minimize stiffness, maximize range of motion, and prevent further compensatory problems down the line.

Hold the stretch for 30-60 seconds. You want to give plenty of time for the muscle to respond appropriately. Tighter muscles will need a longer stretch.

The Take-Home Message:

- Incorporate some form of aerobic exercise, strength training, and stretching every week.
- Shoot for a minimum of 30 minutes of aerobic exercise at your fitness level, three times per week.

- Shoot for a minimum of two strength training sessions per week at 15 minutes each.
- Either do some stretching after every workout, or make it a practice to attend a yoga, pilates, or Tai chi class once or twice a week.

Chapter 14

Building Block #6: Recreation

One man's recreation is another man's work.

Personally I can't stand Sudoku (probably because I am not very good with number puzzles). I'm not a big fan of crossword puzzles, either. But I know several people who think both are very relaxing. I have patients who despise all forms of exercise, yet I have others who participate in bodybuilding competitions for the sheer pleasure of it. Some of my friends think of cooking as a chore, and others are gourmet chefs, regularly hosting dinner parties in their spare time.

But here's the question. What do you spend most of your time doing? Does it recharge you, or deplete you? And if it depletes you, what (if anything) are you doing to refuel?

Many people now struggle with ADT, or Attention Deficit Trait—a product of our fast-paced environment. Due to high-pressure, noisy work environments requiring multitasking in order to get anything done, these people increasingly find it difficult to prioritize, stay organized, and manage their time effectively. Some of the problems associated with ADT are decreased productivity, insomnia, anxiety, irritability, and fatigue—particularly adrenal fatigue (which comes from long term stress; see Chapter 5).

Activity that habitually "depletes" you is stressful by definition. One of the most important mediators for stress due to overwork is to take at least 24 consecutive hours off from what you consider "work" every week, and choose instead to do what you consider "fun."

Taking a "Sabbath" Rest

This concept is not new. One of, if not the earliest, mentions of it showed up in Judaic law (what is now the Old Testament in Christianity), requiring the Jews to take 24 hours off of work every Saturday, from sun up to sun down. Prior to this time, the Jews had been enslaved by the Egyptians for 400 years, during which time they worked 7 days a week, 365 days a year. Originally the Sabbath was meant to be a gift to them, enabling them to rest without feeling guilty for "slacking off."

But by the time Jesus showed up, the religious leaders had attached many additional rules to what did and did not constitute "work," making the Sabbath into a chore, rather than a true day of rest. Jesus (angrily) told them they were totally missing the spirit of the command—God intended to save them from the overwork from which He had originally delivered them.

The point is, rest looks different for everyone. But the ultimate goal is to recharge from life's depleting effects, so that we can return to our regular world and act more effectively than before.

Obviously, sleep is one of the best ways to recharge. Getting enough sleep is fundamental, but it's amazing how often we manage to convince ourselves that we don't really need it that much. Hopefully Chapter 12 convinced you otherwise. We need a good night's sleep—every night.

You can also replenish yourself by enjoying what you've worked for! One of my favorite handouts to give patients was inspired by Stephen Covey's "7 Habits of Highly Effective People," and it is the "urgent vs important" chart.[1] It's a tool to help differentiate between those activities that are truly important (meaning the consequences of not doing them will be severe) versus those activities that are merely urgent (meaning people are yelling at us to do them ASAP —or we are yelling at ourselves—but it really won't matter that much in the long run if we let them slide.) Activities that fall under the "not urgent but important" category are those that allow us to develop the life we truly desire to lead. They are things like enjoying family and friends, engaging in hobbies we love, getting healthy, and serving others. These are the activities that refuel us, rather than deplete us. But because they're not "urgent," many of us will ignore them… and then wonder why life doesn't look the way we wish it did.

Have some unstructured time. This is time to do whatever you feel like doing, and it will be different for each person. It's most restorative to take 24 consecutive hours off every week; without it, you can predispose yourself to illness the following week (because chronic stress depletes the immune system). I give this "prescription" to my Type A patients who approach life from the perspective that "there's always more to do!" They are right, there is always more that could be done—and this is the very reason why it's so important to prioritize time off. Work will always expand to fill however much time you give it. (I know this first-hand!)

Finding a hobby can be critical if you dislike your job, or find it draining. What do you love to do? What would you have done if other "practical" concerns hadn't gotten in the way? This doesn't necessarily have to be a side project, though it can be. If you are an extreme extrovert and you have a desk job that allows for little social interaction, this might look like intentionally cultivating more interpersonal time. If you are an introvert and you are in sales or something that requires lots of face time with others (or if you're a parent and you're with the kids all day long), this might mean intentionally setting aside time to be alone.

Smiling and laughing is a great way to recharge. There is always the "chicken or the egg" question when it comes to mood—are you sad because your "happy" neurotransmitters are low, or are your neurotransmitters low because you are sad? Either way, the evidence shows that your facial expression not only reflects your mood, but also influences it.[2] Smiling and laughing make you feel happier, even if at first you only do it out of sheer willpower. (Caveat here, though: this does not mean you should suppress your negative emotions, as suppression can be dangerous. It just means you should not wallow in them. More on this in Chapter 16.)

There are Seasons for Everything

I realize it isn't always possible to take a full 24 hours off, or to take evenings off all the time. If you're building a new business, you will probably have to put in a lot of extra hours. If you're in a demanding graduate school, you probably won't have a vibrant social life (or if you do, you probably won't do too well in school!) If you've got a toddler at home with special needs, it might be a few years before you can really take much time for yourself.

The key is recognizing within yourself whether your season of intense work with little downtime has turned into a lifestyle. This can easily occur, especially if that period of intense work has gone on long enough to turn into a habit. We've conditioned ourselves to think, "If I don't put in those extra hours, someone else at the office will get the promotion!", or "If I just work a little longer, I'll get X many new clients, which will translate into more money, more security, or more prestige" …or even, "If I don't continue to put in overtime, I might lose my job, and then who will feed my family?"

It takes wisdom to navigate these situations. You probably know within yourself whether you have turned a season of overwork into a lifestyle of overwork. If you don't know, consider asking someone you trust (and who does not have a vested interest in the answer) whether they believe you have done this and if it's time to begin setting some boundaries.

Rest is Productive!

If you are chronically overworked, you will almost certainly notice an increase in your productivity when you listen to the cry of your body and your mind for rest, recreation, and fun. Often, mild cases of insomnia and anxiety, digestive disturbances, tension headaches, irritability and the like will spontaneously resolve with a little R&R. If this is you, take it as your body's cue that you're overdoing it. Time to cut back.

According to the LA Times, over 50% of Americans go more than a year without a vacation (defined as a week off of work, and more than 100 miles from home).[3] This is the lowest percentage in *four decades*. Surveys have found that this is because workers fear they'll be considered expendable if they take time off, because they're gunning for a promotion, because they fear the avalanche of work upon their return, or because they think no one else can do their job while they're gone.

According to Time Magazine, of those who do go on vacation, 61% of us still do some work while we're supposed to be relaxing![4] In this day and age of constant connectivity, it's hard to completely unplug. But working long hours and skipping vacations can have disastrous health effects.

The famous Framingham Study shows that homemakers who take a vacation from being stay-at-home moms every 6 years or less (because let's face it, most of them take their kids with them wherever they go) have twice the risk of heart attacks compared to those who vacation twice per year or more.[5] Also, regular work days of 10 + hours increase the risk of heart attack by 80% in both sexes.[6]

Unless you really love your job, long grueling days tend to sap your joy and make you more prone to anxiety and meltdowns. Compared to those who worked a normal 7-8 hour day, those who regularly work 11-hour shifts have twice the risk of major depression.[7]

Case Study:

Henrietta came to me with periodic severe abdominal cramping, and fatigue so crushing that she sometimes had to pull over when she drove, for fear that she might wreck. We spent most of the first visit talking about her job: she was a music teacher in a dangerous part of town, under an excessively harsh administration. She worked very long hours, took her work home with her, and felt powerless as her bosses continually demanded more. "But there isn't much demand for music teachers," she told me. "What else can I do? Where else can I go?"

For several visits we simply chased symptoms, with small gains. Finally I told Henrietta a personal story from my own family: years ago, my dad's job was thankless and demanded long hours. He worked long days and many nights until wee hours.

At the height of his stress, he was diagnosed with pancreatic cancer. Two weeks later, he was gone.

I warned Henrietta not to let her job take more from her than she was willing to give.

For whatever reason, that story hit home. Henrietta applied for other jobs, and within a few months, she found one. She had to move to take it, but she's never been happier. The abdominal cramping vanished, and the fatigue completely resolved. For the first time in as long as she could remember, Henrietta said she was doing things she enjoyed, and she looks forward to getting up in the morning.

If declining mental health wasn't bad enough, working too much makes you less intelligent, too! The Whitehall II Study study shows that reasoning and creativity drops as work weeks climb above 55 hours.[8] That makes sense, right? Long hours make it harder to think clearly.

The message here, obviously, is to take a vacation. But in order to maximize its restorative capacity, don't always choose one like lounging on the beach. Vacations involving learning new skills are especially good for recharging your batteries.[9]

So consider learning a new skill! Take cooking classes. Go on a yoga retreat. Learn to surf or ski. Pick up a new language. Learn to paint. Have an adventure you can take home with you!

And Now, For Some Perspective

Your recreational time is bound to include social functions or family get-togethers: moments you want to enjoy but may be spending with people who do not share your lifestyle. Different diets and lifestyles are normal and need not create stress in what would otherwise be a fun, relaxing situation. Here, too, the key is balance.

When I was a naturopathic medical student, I was surrounded by other students who shared my healthy nutritional lifestyle. Once I graduated and rejoined the rest of the population socially, I realized that I couldn't be dogmatic anymore—particularly about my food choices, because so many social activities involve food. If I insisted on eating only unprocessed whole foods free of trans fats, chemicals, and added sugar, the people around me would feel judged, even if I didn't consciously intend it. But on the other hand, I didn't want to compromise my health, and I knew too much to think it truly wouldn't make a difference in the long run.

It helps to try and think about it from the other person's perspective. Many younger people who haven't lived long enough to accumulate much damage tend to give almost no thought to nutrition. Making healthy food choices can be more expensive and require self-discipline. As long as they feel healthy, why go to such effort for no apparent gain?

Even some older adults disregard nutrition as long as symptoms are relatively mild and decently controlled with medications. It might not seem like a big deal to have that soda with a meal, or even to choose the salad dressing that has sugar listed as its second ingredient. Of course, it adds up—on average, every American consumes nearly 156 pounds of added sugar per year.[10] But in the moment, what's one more dessert? For most people, it isn't until their symptoms have become very severe indeed that they're willing to consider the impact of their lifestyle choices on their health. Until then, the benefits of change just don't appear to be worth the sacrifice. This is very human: most of us will resist change until the moment when the pain of changing becomes lower than the pain of staying the same. (I'll bet you can identify at least one negative area in your own life where you're resisting change for exactly this reason.)

But on the flip side, our bodies are amazingly resilient for the most part. If you're generally conscious about your health, and you're blessed with a constitution that is not highly sensitive, then one soda, one sugary condiment or one extra dessert won't have a severe impact. Like anything else, it's a cost/benefit analysis. Is sticking to your diet or your principles worth offending your dinner host? Unless you have a serious restriction (i.e. you have Celiac disease and they're serving pizza), in my opinion the answer is generally no. I don't feel great after I eat junk food either, so I try not to do it if I can help it. But sometimes the social capital is more important—provided I'm not in a position to make that compromise too regularly.

The Take-Home Message:

- **Take vacations.** At least once a year, for heaven's sake.
- **Schedule at least 24 hours off every week.** That means you're only allowed to do things you enjoy during that time, only things that recharge you. They don't have to be a consecutive 24 hours, although if you can manage that I would highly recommend it. Consecutive time off is much more restorative than a little here, a little there.
- **Make time for things you love!** These should actually get scheduled into your week, if you're a workaholic. That way you'll actually do them.
- **Try not to be too rigid,** for you perfectionists out there. It's good to eat healthy most of the time, of course! But if you're invited to a party and you know they'll be serving take-out pizza, unless you have major health reasons why you shouldn't, go and have a slice. (If you want to, of course.) Or if you do have major health reasons why you shouldn't, then eat something at home first, and still go!

Chapter 15

BUILDING BLOCK #7:
SOLID RELATIONSHIPS

H ealthy relationships can be defined by two general rules:

1. We must be able to share with another person (or group of people) who we really are—flaws and all.
2. The other person (or group) must be willing to love and accept us as we are, without criticism or judgment.

But obviously it doesn't always happen quite like that. If we engage in #1, we open ourselves up to the possibility of rejection or loss if the other person or the community fails to exercise #2. That happens to all of us at some point.

If we've internalized enough acceptance and connection over time, though, we can handle rejection or loss and still continue to offer our true selves in other relationships in the future. But if we haven't, eventually we shut down emotionally. Shutting down precludes enjoying new, healing relationships—because of course, we have to be willing to show others who we are before they can decide whether or not to love us.

There are many disabling behaviors that indicate a pattern of shutting down; these are the ones I encounter most frequently in my practice. See if you recognize yourself in any of them.

Addictions happen when we use a surrogate to try and fill a real need—and we can use almost anything (including substances, shopping, gambling, sex, and food. For instance, ever found yourself craving sugar and white carbs around mid-afternoon or the evening, especially when you're depressed or feeling down? If so, you are likely self-medicating: these foods help our bodies to produce the neurotransmitter serotonin). You might have an addiction if you seek a surrogate like one of these to relieve negative emotions, especially if you never feel like you've had enough of it. Another red flag might be if one of these surrogates consumes a lot of your resources (mentally, emotionally, financially, or physically). Jesus said in Luke 12:34, "For where your treasure is, there will your heart be also."

Self-sufficiency says, "I don't need you anyway." It might start out looking like sour grapes, but over time it moves into true denial of the need for other people. Denial tends to keep us "stuck" and therefore isolated, because obviously if we don't realize we need others, we're not about to open up to them (which means it's impossible for us to receive what we really need from them—their love).

Perfectionism. The logic tends to be, "If I were only more (fill in the blank), then they would love me." The trouble is, perfectionists can never relax. Every compliment sounds to their ears like an expectation to do even better the next time. There is usually a lot of fear surrounding the idea that at some point, others will find out who they really are, and they will lose love as a result.

People-pleasing. People pleasers tend to be chameleons; who they are, what they like, and what they will or won't tolerate depends on whom they happen to be with at the time. They often have a hard time saying no, fearing that setting limits will provoke anger and thus, lose love.

If you've adopted protective mechanisms, you've adopted them for a reason. They're symptoms, telling you that there's a problem hiding underneath that still needs to be healed. One of the primary tenets of naturopathic medicine is to *treat the root cause, rather than the symptom.* If you try to discipline yourself to kick your addiction, or to stop wanting admiration, or to stop putting so much pressure on yourself, you'll only be frustrated. If the underlying reason for those protective mechanisms hasn't been addressed, willpower simply won't work. The instinct for self-preservation is too strong.

What does work, in a word, is grace. Only the first of the two conditions for healthy relationships depends upon us (sharing who we really are), but we must do our part. We have to risk showing our less-than-perfect sides to safe people. It's important to choose someone with whom to share who is not likely to be overly critical—support groups or churches are a great place to start. When you've internalized enough love and acceptance from safe relationships, life's inevitable losses and rejections will be much easier to take and you will be more comfortable seeking relationships in the future.

Some people, on the other hand, are relationship seekers by nature. If they have not established the habits and attitudes that are necessary for healthy, functional relationships, they soon end up feeling misunderstood, unappreciated, and, often, trapped. This feeling of powerlessness in a relationship arises from an inability to find the balance we seek. Specifically, we feel powerless when we don't think we can say no without suffering some consequence (damaging a relationship, losing a job, feeling guilty, etc). We desperately desire a particular outcome that we believe is outside our control, or we don't see any way out of a negative or toxic environment, either at work or home or elsewhere.

Feeling Powerless

The biggest power issue I tend to see in my practice (and one I've struggled with myself!) is guilt. "Isn't it selfish to say no when I could say yes?" we ask.

On one hand, helping others is one of the most fulfilling experiences in life. It is good to look out for the interests of others, and not just for our own. If we have the resources to help, and we want to help, then we should help.

But that "want to" is key—the whole thing hinges on the concept of choice. **In order to say yes from your heart, you first have to have the ability to say no.** If you don't feel like "no" is an option, then a "yes" can only come from compulsion (not from love). If you find yourself frequently saying yes when you want to say no, you are not actually being selfless—you're being hypocritical.

The Apostle Paul says that we should each give "what [we have] decided in [our hearts] to give, not reluctantly or under compulsion, for God loves a cheerful giver" (2 Corinthians 9:7). Saying "yes" when you really mean "no" breeds resentment, and can cause you to withdraw from a person who makes demands (the "passive aggressive" approach), which damages relationships far more than simply saying what you mean. Over time this sort of disconnect between who you really are and who you present yourself to be can also lead to problems with anxiety. (Remember, emotions are symptoms of a problem, and not the problem itself!)

A prerequisite for any healthy relationship is freedom. So let your "yes be yes, and your no be no" (Matthew 5:37).

Case Study:

Alice came to me with hot flashes, fatigue, weight gain, and IBS—the typical constellation of symptoms. But no matter how I tried, I couldn't get her to stick to the description of physical symptoms. What she wanted to talk about was how powerless she felt in her life. Her daughter-in-law manipulated and controlled her, and she didn't feel like she could stand up to her for fear of losing her son. Besides, wasn't it selfish for her to refuse to help with her grandkids just as much as her daughter-in-law wanted?

We spent most of the first visit discussing boundaries. I did give her a lab requisition to see about any physical causes of her symptoms and sent her home with a diet diary, but her real homework was to read "Boundaries" by Henry Cloud and John Townsend, and get it clear in her mind that rather than standing in the way of a real relationship, her 'no' would enable a real relationship to be a possibility. Even if her daughter-in-law and perhaps her son reacted in anger, her health was suffering as a result of her poor boundaries and refusal to care for herself.

It turned out Alice did have very low hormones, hypothyroidism, and a poor diet, so we addressed all of those things. But the real turning point came when she told me, with a big grin, that at last she had set some limits. Much to her surprise, they were well-received! She felt much closer to her family afterwards, she was sleeping better, her energy returned, she'd started exercising, she was eating better, her gut symptoms vanished, and she was losing weight. She told me how much more peaceful she felt once she'd become a peace maker, rather than a people pleaser.

It is important to keep in mind, however, that even if you are agreeing to something that comes easily from your heart, there is always the possibility that although you have the ability to help, you shouldn't. Newton's Third Law of Motion says, "For every action, there's an equal and opposite reaction." In the same way, there are also consequences for our actions in life. Good consequences are reinforcing—they teach us, "Hey, I want more where that came from, so I'll keep on doing what I did to get it!" while bad consequences teach us, "Well, that stunk. Better not do that again."

There's an apparent exception to this rule, though: you can step in and shoulder the consequences for someone else's actions, and circumvent the process. Most of us will agree on a moral basis that it's not okay to steal the positive rewards of someone else's labor. But there's disagreement over whether shielding someone we love from the negative consequences of his or her poor choices is a "loving" thing to do.

What it comes down to is this. If the person you love recognizes that he has made poor choices and is sorry, then he's not as likely to make a similar choice in the future. In that case, shielding him from the consequences may be loving—as long as you want to, have the resources to do so, and haven't already bailed him out multiple times in the past!

However, if the person you love does not recognize that he has made a poor choice, by shielding him from the consequences, you are preventing him from learning from it. That's called enabling. Proverbs 19:19 says, "A hot-tempered man must pay the penalty; if you rescue him, you will have to do it again." It's best to let this kind of person reap what he sows, and learn the hard way.

Case Study:

Lilian had a son on drugs, who had become homeless because of his addiction. She told me that for a long time, she and her husband had done everything they could to "rescue" him—paying his rent so he wouldn't be homeless, giving him money, bringing him groceries, nagging him to clean up his life. But finally she had a frank conversation with a youth pastor who told her, "The only way your son is going to change, the only chance he has, is if you stop enabling him. Then he'll either crash and burn, or he'll turn around. But until then, he hasn't had to face any consequences for his behavior. He has no reason to change."

Lilian and her husband listened. She told me the one thing she insisted on doing was continuing to bring him groceries, because she couldn't bear the thought of him going hungry. But they allowed him to become homeless. They stopped giving him money. They stopped nagging.

While their son is still rebellious, he's made strides that have indicated he's waking up—in fact, he's held a job consistently for the first time in years! Meanwhile, Lilian has recovered her peace, and her health.

For more on all of these concepts, I highly recommend the book "Boundaries" by Henry Cloud and John Townsend.[1] I recommend it to patients all the time!

Emotional Freedom

Saying what you mean and understanding that it is not your responsibility to bear the consequences of another's actions will go far in preventing a situation of powerlessness. Sometimes, despite our efforts to create and sustain balance with boundaries and personal responsibility, we end up in a relationship that simply feels as if it will suck the life right out of us. These energy drainers can come in the form of difficult people or of unwanted circumstances. When faced with an energy drainer, there are essentially three ways you can respond: you can change the situation; you can change yourself so that the situation becomes tolerable; or you can leave the situation.

It takes wisdom to identify which of the three is appropriate. It's never possible to change another person (and if you try, you're almost guaranteed to make the problem worse). But you might be able to set limits on a person, by saying, "If you continue to speak to me harshly, I will not continue to associate with you." This does not change the other person; she can continue to be rude if she likes, but you won't be around to hear it. In that case, you have changed the situation. And this is not selfish: remember, we are not responsible for another person's needs, desires, or feelings. We can help as we want to and as we are able, but ultimately the needs, desires, and feelings of others are all their responsibility.

If you aren't in a position to set limits, consider re-framing the way you view the situation. Maybe the inefficiency of your coworkers becomes an opportunity for you to exercise patience. Maybe you can de-escalate a conflict by deciding to stay calm, rather than reacting with anger. We don't have control over other people, and we don't always have control over our circumstances, but we do have control over ourselves.

There are times when it's appropriate to cut your losses, though. Abuse of any kind is never acceptable, but it takes support from others to leave a toxic relationship, to walk away from an overly demanding job, or to withdraw from an important person. You definitely need spiritual and emotional support in order to make such a major change in your life, so make sure you find a good support group of friends, family, or other like-minded people who will be there for you through difficult times.

Stop and Evaluate

If you constantly feel worn out, I'd highly encourage you to identify the energy drainers in your life. Sit down in a quiet place with a pen and paper and write out your sources of stress. When you identify the biggest one or the biggest several, see which of the three approaches (change the situation, change yourself, or leave) is most appropriate. Cultivate the support you need to keep you accountable and help you through (including a qualified counselor if you feel that is necessary)... and then take the steps you need to take to help you regain power over your life.

Unfortunately, sometimes life is just stressful, and there's nothing you can do about it. In those situations, all we can do is take good care of ourselves and learn good stress management techniques. I highly recommend beginning a spiritual practice if you do not have one already. Prayer has a way of grounding us, and reminding us that even though we may not be in control of a situation, there is One who is in control, and who is on our side. Journaling also really helps to get some of those spinning thoughts down on paper, and helping you to make sense of your emotions—often this alone functions as an excellent stress management technique! I also love meditation, yoga, regular exercise especially in nature, and scheduling time to do things you enjoy. For more on stress management options, see Chapter 16.

Most of us tend to assume there's nothing we can do about our stress, even when that isn't the case. You just learned about identifying your energy drainers and sorting them into one of three categories: *things you can change, things you can refuse to tolerate, or things you can (or must) choose to accept.*

One of those stressors I hear about over and over in my practice is taking responsibility for other people's happiness. If you find that you are held captive by someone else's emotions, the first question to ask yourself is whether the person in question is a safe person, or an emotional vampire.

Emotional vampires are those who tend to suck you dry (pun fully intended—and no, I did not coin the term emotional vampires, but I wish I did). They may criticize, try to control or otherwise manipulate you. Sometimes your relationships with other people will suffer because of your relationship with them. If you feel responsible for the happiness of an emotional vampire, this kind of stressor needs to fall under the category of "things you refuse to tolerate." Nobody can force you to accept poor treatment, and nobody can emotionally manipulate you without your consent. If the relationship is unavoidable, then drawing firm and appropriate boundaries with that person is absolutely essential. Remember that *what you put up with, you end up with.*

Safe people, on the other hand, are accepting, forgiving, kind, honest, and help you to become your best self. They are "for" you. Nobody can be this way 100% of the time, of course, because we're all human—but if you tend to feel responsible for the emotions of a generally safe individual, then this falls under the category of "things you can change"—about yourself.

If you're a people pleaser, you probably don't feel right when you think someone is mad at you. That's normal—nobody likes it when someone is upset with them. And it is important that we strive to live at peace with others, so far as it depends upon us (Romans 12:18). The appropriate way to deal with a legitimate breach in a relationship is to approach the other person directly and have a conversation about it. Safe people will welcome honesty and directness, and most likely this approach will strengthen the relationship.

But if you're always thinking people are upset with you even when they're not, or if you find that your emotional well-being is contingent upon someone else's happiness, that's called codependency. Codependency is taking responsibility for something that is rightfully another person's problem, or allowing someone else to take responsibility for something that is rightfully yours.

Remember that control and responsibility go together: if it's under your control, it's probably your responsibility. If it's not under your control, then it would be pretty ridiculous to hold yourself responsible for it. Specifically, *your needs, desires, and feelings are your responsibility, while the needs, desires, and feelings of others are theirs.*

One important note here: even if you *can* give the other person what they want and you think this will make them happy, it is not your *responsibility* to do so (provided the relationship is a personal one, and not based upon employment or some other type of agreed-upon compensation).

Remember to stand your ground. If the other person doesn't like it, it's not your problem—it's theirs!

For more emotionally healthy individuals, simply identifying your destructive patterns may be enough to help you conquer them. But if you have a history of trauma, you may require professional counseling to help unravel codependent tendencies. Either way, recognizing the pattern is a huge first step towards emotional freedom and healthy relationships. Attaining both is beneficial not only for your mental health, but also for your physical health and may ultimately have an impact on your longevity.

The Surprising Benefit of Healthy Relationships

Notably, longevity researchers have discovered that, in general, centenarians are often described as likable. Perhaps this has something to do with the fact that happiness is contagious.[2] We like to be around people who are happy because they make us happy too. As a result, these happy, likable centenarians, who are genuinely compassionate and interested in other people, are relationship experts. They tend to get better care from their caregivers and also have a greater social support system, the importance of which cannot be overestimated.

In Malcolm Gladwell's book *Outliers,* he highlights the concentration of centenarians in the little Italian immigrant community of Roseto, Pennsylvania in 1961. The community had rates of heart disease half that of the national average at the time, and nearly zero for men under 65—as well as a death rate 30-35% lower than the national average for all causes.[3] A professor of the University of Oklahoma Medical School wanted to find out why. To his surprise, he discovered that the people of Roseto had a diet that was far from healthy, they got very little exercise, and their Italian relatives in other parts of the U.S. enjoyed no similar protection (so they didn't have their genes to thank). But something else also set them apart from the national norm: community living and multigenerational homes. Neighbors strolled the streets together in the evenings. They went to church together. They had dinner together. Their children played together. They looked out for each other.

A generation later, the "old ways" began to change as the younger generation in Roseto grew up and moved away, and the very close-knit community life the immigrants had enjoyed began to disintegrate. Over the next decade, heart disease in Roseto doubled, hypertension tripled, and the rate of fatal heart attacks reached the national average by the end of the 1970s.

It turned out that what kept that idyllic community healthy was the community itself.

The Take-Home Message:

Healthy relationships are important—not only for your quality of life, but also for your health. If you're not already plugged into a community, make it a priority to seek one out. Find a community of like-minded individuals. A great place to try out is a church, and particularly a small group or a Bible study within a church. These groups are small enough that it's still possible to get to know people within them, and have a common faith to bring them together. Churches are excellent places to find those whose desire is to "do life together."

Another option I love is meetup.com. You can search on this website for any hobby you happen to fancy, and find groups of other individuals who share your interest—from hiking to knitting to philosophy discussions to ethnic cuisine. Sign up to receive emails of when and where they plan to meet next. If you can't find a meetup group that matches your interest, you can start one! Anyone who has indicated an interest in the keywords you use to describe your group will receive an email alert that the group has been created, and an invitation to join.

You also might consider taking a continuing education class. Remember college—how easy it was to just meet your classmates and form study groups that turned into friendships? This might be a way to recreate that. If you're older and you're looking at a local university or community college for this, you probably would want to make sure that the course you chose was listed as "continuing education" or "non-degree seeking," to make it more likely that there might be others in a similar life stage to yours among the students.

Chapter 16

BUILDING BLOCK #8: PEACE
AND A SENSE OF PURPOSE

ccording to psychologist Abraham Maslow, mankind attempts to meet his needs in a particular hierarchy. First, he will meet his physiological needs— those functions necessary for immediate survival. Once those needs have been attended to, he will meet his need for security, ensuring that his survival needs will be met for the future. After that, he will meet his need for community— that is, love and friendship. Then he will attend to his self-perception, including achievement of personal goals and respect from others.

But even once these needs are met, the final crowning desire is for self-actualization, or reaching his highest potential.[1] According to the author of the biblical Proverbs (27:20), no one ever fully realizes it in this life, and this is as it must be: consider the men who walked on the moon or won Olympic golds and then fell into despair after the fact, having nothing higher to achieve. The point is the process. So, if you've climbed Maslow's ladder and currently linger somewhere between self-perception and self-actualization, what comes next?

Finding Purpose

I found nuggets of wisdom addressing this question in Timothy Ferriss's *The Four Hour Work Week*.[2] Assuming you have the luxury of time to devote to this question, this is what he has to say on the subject:

First do nothing. This is absolutely necessary, because modern life is loud. If we want to hear anything other than external noise, we have to choose it consciously. The purpose of this is to tune in, and learn to make the distinction between your inner voice and the opinions and ideas of the world around you. Be warned, though: this is scary. Silence has a way of bringing up deep questions and fears. If silence is completely out of your comfort zone, just start with a few minutes per day of breathing quietly and tuning in, expanding the length of time gradually as you become more comfortable with the process.

> **Personal story here:** during one of my quarter breaks in medical school, I decided to take my own five-day fasting and meditation retreat, even though I didn't go anywhere. The goal was to really get quiet before God and tune in to whatever He might be trying to communicate to me. I watched no TV or movies, I didn't schedule any social activities, and I didn't read any books except scripture. I journaled, and I got out into nature… a lot.
>
> It was HARD. I started going stir-crazy within the first 12 hours. I got depressed, and found it almost impossible to focus my mind on any one thing for any length of time. I started to realize that I was essentially going through withdrawals, from the constant activity and stimuli in my life.
>
> By the third day, the restlessness passed. Nothing extraordinary happened on the other end of that retreat externally—but I can say that some key areas in my mindset shifted. My mind quieted down. My trust in God deepened. My purpose didn't exactly solidify, but it grew much clearer than it had been before. I also learned how loud my life was,

and how distracted I had been as a baseline. I've been able to carry that awareness forward, checking in with myself at various points to see if I'm becoming distracted and unfocused, and attempting to realign myself with where I want to be.

Recognize that we are designed to problem-solve. Even when our lives are going well for the most part, left to our own devices, we all have a tendency to focus on what still needs fixing. Don't beat yourself up about it, but don't become a victim either. In his book, *Learned Optimism*, Martin Seligman describes a cohort of clinically depressed patients whose only treatment was a daily gratitude journal, which served to shift their focus from the problems still to be solved to the blessings that had been solved already. The result? Ninety-four percent of them reported subjective improvement in their depressive symptoms within a month.[3] The point is, when you get quiet, your mind will naturally gravitate towards the problems in your life. Be conscious of this and redirect those thoughts.

Choose an ambitious goal. The answer to fulfillment is bigger than just gratitude: if we learn to appreciate where we are, all we've done is override the natural bent of our minds to (as Ferriss writes) "turn inward on itself and create problems for us to solve, even if the problems are undefined or unimportant." The solution Ferriss proposes is to choose some seemingly impossible goal that resonates with us. Once we've identified the goal, we start moving towards it. Now our focus is "out there." We are energized and focused. We have purpose.

Most of the time when we talk about such elusive concepts as "self-esteem," this is what we're really discussing. The word self-esteem can be misleading, though, because purpose usually resides outside of ourselves. It has to do with how we can contribute to the well-being of others, how we can make the world a better place, or how we can help to support and care for those we love.

In Viktor Frankl's book, *Man's Search for Meaning*, this Jewish psychiatrist who survived the concentration camps writes, "This uniqueness and singleness which distinguishes each individual and gives a meaning to his existence has a bearing on creative work as much as it does on human love. When the impossibility of replacing a person is realized, it allows the responsibility which a man has for his existence and its continuance to appear in all its magnitude. A man who becomes conscious of the responsibility he bears toward a human being who affectionately waits for him, or to an unfinished work, will never be able to throw away his life. He knows the 'why' for his existence, and will be able to bear almost any 'how.'" According to Frankl, the pursuit of happiness is the wrong focus; happiness results from having and fulfilling one's purpose. Or to quote Frankl again, "What man actually needs is not a tensionless state but rather a striving and struggling for a worthwhile goal, a freely chosen task." [4]

Obviously, having a purpose is imperative, but you may have more than one single purpose. I've always wondered what happens to the hero of an adventure story after the story ends… if the quest consumed his whole life, his prospects after the fact seem pretty bleak. It is very common for people whose jobs or parenthood largely define them to suffer from depression after retirement, or when the kids leave home. But remember…. if you're still here, you still have more to do. How many things are on your 'bucket list'? How many causes are you passionate about? How many talents have you yet to fully develop?

If you cannot answer these questions, start with step one… get quiet. Do nothing, stick with it, and wait for the answers to come.

Take Inventory

Part of waiting for the answers to come is to stop and take inventory of your life. How's it working out for you? Are you happy with not only where you are now, but with where you are headed in the major areas of your life (your relationships, your finances, your job, and your health—all aspects of it)?

If not, here's a exercise, called the One Page Miracle (I borrowed this from Dr. Amen, author of *Change Your Brain, Change Your Life*).[5] It goes like this:

Separate your life into those four major categories (Relationships, Work, Money, Myself). Then break each category down further into subcategories.

For example, under relationships, if you are married, put spouse/partner, as well as children if you have them, extended family, and friends. Then write down a specific, measurable goal for the next year in each of those subcategories. (For instance, "I would like to call my adult children once a week," or "I would like to plan and schedule a date night with my husband once a week.") Here's your template:

RELATIONSHIPS
- **Spouse/Partner:**
- **Children:**
- **Extended Family:**
- **Friends:**

"Work" is whatever you spend most of your time doing. If you are a stay-at-home mom, then it will overlap with the relationship section, but it will include things like teaching your children how to play well with others, and planning time to shower every day while they're napping (I know that can be a challenge sometimes!) If you have multiple jobs, or a job and an important hobby, that goes here too. If you volunteer, that goes here. Again, make sure what you write down is specific, actionable, and measurable—"what gets measured gets improved," after all.

WORK
- **My job:**
- **My hobby:**
- **Volunteering:**

"Money" should be broken down into short term and long term goals. I recommend breaking the short term goal down to a fiscal quarter (three months) while the long-term goal should be more where you'd like to be financially within the next year. If you're in debt, perhaps the goal could be to pay down a certain amount of your credit card bill each month, and put a certain amount in savings.

MONEY
- **Short term:**
- **Long term:**

Under "myself", you should include body, mind, and spirit, since we are comprised of all three. Most people's goals tend to focus only on the first, but true health means all of the above, and is heavily influenced by the quality of our relationships, work, and finances. It's impossible to be truly healthy without maintaining order in all of those categories.

So for your body, consider resolutions to eat healthier, exercise more, drink more water, take your vitamins, and get enough sleep... as well as perhaps to minimize any health-related addiction you may battle (alcohol, soda, smoking, overeating, too much sugar, etc). This latter point may require accountability from others to keep you honest.

Let's lump thoughts and emotions together under 'mind.' These goals may include cultivating a positive body image (especially as a counterbalance to some of the weight-loss goals in the body category), finding and pursuing a new interest to keep you intellectually stimulated, being kinder to yourself, playing more, or eliminating your "energy suckers."

And spirit involves connection with a higher power. I have certainly found that many "energy suckers" in the mind category must be dealt with on a spiritual level. A solid belief in a God who cares for you and acts positively on your behalf is a critical ingredient for deep healing from old wounds and getting out of our own way on the road to happiness and fulfillment. If you don't have a spiritual belief system or practice that is meaningful and important to your life, this is the time to start.

MYSELF
- **Body:**
- **Mind:**
- **Spirit:**

All of this should fit into a single page so that it's simple, direct, and actionable. In order for this exercise to be as effective as possible, keep your page in a place where you can see it every day. This will remind you going forward to make choices in keeping with your goals, and will make it much more likely that you will actually achieve them.

Dealing With Indecision

You may find yourself struggling with indecision when making some of the choices that will put you on the path to achieving your goals. This indecision is one of our biggest sources of stress and anxiety. My approach to this one, and the approach I teach my patients, is a step-wise process based on biblical teaching. Again, if the Bible doesn't resonate with you, glean what you can and keep what you can agree with. The process can still help you.

Give it to God

The first step is to realize that you are not in control anyway—that is an illusion. Think back over the events in your life: list the other times that you have tried to control your circumstances.

Did it work? What was the outcome?

Most of the time, if we're honest, we know that the answer to this is no. Sometimes we think we're in control, but we all have plenty of stories in our lives that prove this isn't ultimately the case. Admit that you are powerless to make your life work out the way you want it to. As long as you're in denial about that, you'll stay stuck. "Many are the plans in a man's heart, but it is the Lord's purpose that prevails" (Proverbs 19:21).

After you realize that you are not in control, acknowledge that God wants to be first in your life. This is the key to defeating control and anxiety: we are anxious when we want something more than we want to follow God. Letting go of the thing we desire is terrifying (in fact, it feels a lot like dying to ourselves), but it is the only path to peace. The paradox is, God promises that if we lose our life, that is when we will find it. As long as we insist on controlling our lives, it will remain forever out of control. "Seek first his kingdom and his righteousness, and all these things will be given to you as well. Therefore do not worry about tomorrow, for tomorrow will worry about itself. Each day has enough trouble of its own" (Matthew 6:33-34).

When we let go of "trying to find our lives" (whatever the problem is that obsesses us), we will experience grief—but it is a good, healing grief. It is a grief that leads to joy in the end, because it is the only path to life. "Weeping may remain for a night, but rejoicing comes in the morning" (Psalm 30:5).

You must know that while you are experiencing grief, you do not have to bear your pain alone. **God invites you to bring your troubles to Him.** Read his words to remind yourself that he will comfort you. "Come to me, all you who are weary and burdened, and I will give you rest" (Matthew 11:28).

God is a good God; therefore you can trust Him. He is *for* you and not against you; He wants good things for you. "Those who seek the Lord lack no good thing" (Psalm 34:10).

Once you have brought your troubles to God, and prayed for a solution, your job is to do the very hardest thing of all: **wait, and trust that God will do what He said He would do.** "Trust in the Lord with all your heart and lean not on your own understanding; in all your ways acknowledge him and he will make your paths straight" (Proverbs 3:5-6).

But what if you are still supposed to do something to fix the problem? Part of trusting God is trusting that **He will tell you what to do and when to do it (if you are supposed to do anything at all).** That is why we have the Holy Spirit—he promises to guide you into all truth. "I will instruct you and teach you in the way you should go; I will counsel you and watch over you" (Psalm 32:8).

When you act according to the leading of the Holy Spirit, now you are partnering with God and can have faith in the outcome. The Bible defines faith as "the substance of things hoped for; the evidence of things not seen" (Hebrews 11:1). There's a reason why it is called *substance* and *evidence*. Hope is not the same thing as faith; hope is simply a wish or desire, while faith is the belief that the wish will come to pass. You've got to have a reason for faith (while you need none for hope). Faith is the substantive evidence of something that does not yet have physical form. "By his power he may fulfill every good purpose of yours and every act prompted by your faith" (2 Thessalonians 1:11).

The Enemy of Faith: Fear

If you do not have faith, you will have fear. Fear is the substance of things *dreaded*. There is a great deal of power in what you think—not because of metaphysics, but because thoughts become words, and words become actions, and actions bear consequences in our lives, whether good or bad.

Fear has a purpose: it's there to signal impending danger and to warn us to be careful. But it can be blown out of proportion to the actual danger. This is in part because the prefrontal cortex of the human brain is designed to simulate an experience before it happens. This keeps us from having to learn every lesson by hard knocks… but if we choose to imagine every possible negative scenario, no matter how unlikely, then our fear response can be very much exaggerated.

One thing that leads to fear is overgeneralization: we take a single negative event and assume that event will become a pattern. For instance, after a breakup, we conclude, "No one will ever want me. I'll be alone forever." This can become a self-fulfilling prophecy, affecting our choices and the opportunities to which we avail ourselves. (If you think no one will ever want you, how much confidence do you think you're going to give off?)

Labeling also leads to fear: we take a single negative action and generalize it to the person who committed it—ourselves or someone else. For instance, after getting fired, we conclude, "I'm a failure." Or, your spouse does something to hurt you and you conclude, "He is a selfish person." This, too, can become a self-fulfilling prophecy: if you treat someone as selfish, is he more or less likely to be kind to you in the future? If you tell yourself you're a failure, what are the chances you'll take any risks that might lead to success?

Worst-Case-Scenario Thinking: Pessimists usually say that life has taught them to expect the worst. They think they are protecting themselves from disappointment, no matter how unlikely their predictions might be. Proverbs 4:23 says, "Above all else, guard your heart, for it is the wellspring of life." This is because, in reality, pessimists are flooding their bodies with fight-or flight stress hormones, which, over time, can lead to constipation, diarrhea, high blood pressure, high cholesterol, heart disease, diabetes, insomnia, sexual dysfunction, anxiety, immune dysfunction, depression, and even cancer. All this, when more often than not, the things we fear don't even happen!

Fear is a kind of bondage. It is essentially meditation upon something negative instead of upon something positive, which eventually leads to the belief that a negative event will come to pass. If you find that negative thoughts regularly cloud your mind (and your mood), work on recognizing them as they pop up so that you can take a breath, acknowledge the thought, and then release it. Those thoughts do not need to take up residence in your mind.

If you find that you have difficulty with this—and most people do at first—I encourage you to begin a meditation practice.

Mindfulness and Meditation

There are a surprising number of studies that demonstrate the health benefits of meditation—just go to www.pubmed.com, type in meditation, and you'll see what I mean. Even in the mainstream media, mindfulness is catching on as an excellent way to moderate stress.[6]

Meditation and an attitude of mindfulness melt away stress as you learn to reacquaint yourself with the richness of life's details that have gradually begun to escape your notice—your breath, the way your body feels, the beauty and movement of the plants in the wind, or the breeze across your skin. Since beginning meditation, I have noticed that the barrage of thoughts that constantly swirl in my head unacknowledged finally have the ability to surface and have their moment. It's as though they're all petulant children that only want to be given a bit of attention, and that alone is sufficient to calm them down. After that, I can go about my business more peacefully, as if I'm somehow just a bit less susceptible to all matters that aren't immediately pressing.

Start meditating slowly and for a short time. For five minutes, count your breaths up to eight and down again, and allow thoughts to come and go as they may, without fighting them. As you realize you are having a thought, let it go and gently redirect your thoughts back to your breath. Don't beat yourself up: it'll be hard at first, and you'll probably have a lot of thoughts fight for your attention. But it will get easier over time. There are also a number of great apps (if you have a smart phone) that can guide you through this (Headspace is one of my favorites), or YouTube videos on guided meditation that can help to get you started.

Gratitude and Your Overall Health

In his book, *Thanks! How Practicing Gratitude Can Make You Happier,*[7] Robert Emmonds cites that depression and pessimism are linked to shorter life spans. In one study, participants scoring high on optimism had a 55% lower risk of death from all causes than those counted as pessimistic. Another study[8] suggests that the reason for this may be either a direct link between optimism and immune function, and/or a link between optimism and health-promoting activities, such as eating better, exercising, etc. My suspicion is that from a physiologic standpoint, hope, and therefore optimism, decrease levels of harmful stress hormones such as cortisol and adrenaline. Chronically elevated levels of these hormones create cumulative damage.

Gratitude and Depression

In *Thanks!,*[7] Emmond describes one study he conducted over a 10-week period, which randomly assigned its participants into three groups: one group wrote down five things they were grateful for the previous week, one group wrote down five stressors or hassles they'd encountered the previous week, and one group wrote down five neutral events that affected them (without specifying whether the effect was positive or negative). The results? The gratitude group was 25% happier than the other two groups. They also exercised more and reported fewer physical ailments.

Yet another study[9] demonstrates that gratitude is inversely correlated with depression in patients already struggling with chronic illness of arthritis or Irritable Bowel Disease (IBD).

It's well worth your time and effort to take up a daily gratitude practice. I can testify personally to the power this has to redirect my thoughts from sadness to contentment, in the span of only a few moments. I don't know too many other things that can do that!

The Take-Home Message

- **Take inventory**. What are your goals in the major areas of your life: in your relationships, your work, your finances, and your personal growth? Do you feel as if you have a clear purpose, or a set of purposes? If not, get quiet—avoid the external stimuli, get through the withdrawals, and wait for the answers to come.

- **Start meditating**. Getting quiet once is not enough; it needs to become a lifestyle. You can't just set your life course and then expect to reach it without constant course corrections along the way—and one of the blessings of frequent meditations or quiet periods is that it will allow you to recognize when you have gotten off course.

- **Pay attention to your thoughts**. When you are not specifically setting aside time to meditate, you're probably still "meditating," or ruminating, or something. Make sure that your thoughts are both true, and beneficial for you.

- **Keep a gratitude journal.** First thing in the morning or last thing at night, write down five things you're grateful for. (It doesn't have to be five—but that's a good place to start.)

- **Remember where you've come from**. The contrast between where you used to be and where you are now can help you to appreciate the blessings you once lacked, but now enjoy!

- **Record your prayers.** This is a great way to remember where you've come from. It's amazing to see how prayers are answered. So many of us forget that we ever had a need at all after it's been met.

CONCLUSION

I know how you feel.

As a patient myself, I certainly had my work cut out for me. From the time I was fifteen until about halfway through medical school, my gut was so inflamed that I'd forgotten what "normal" felt like. I just assumed everyone felt the way I did!

But there is hope, and healing is possible.

The longer I've been in practice, the more I've come to truly trust in the simplicity of naturopathic medicine. There are only so many building blocks, and there are only so many potential obstacles to cure. Get familiar with those, and it doesn't really matter what the particular disease happens to be called—whether it be IBS, IBD, SIBO, candida overgrowth, mold toxicity, food allergies, you name it—the approach is still quite similar. More often than not, the patient will lead me to the answer we need at the time, if I just ask enough questions and listen well.

But you, the patient, still bear the lion's share of the work. While system imbalances usually do require intervention and guidance from a physician, after that the real work of healing depends upon you. You're the one who will have to avoid those obstacles to cure going forward, and you're the one who must create the environment in which health and healing can prevail.

I hope this guide has helped you to identify your own obstacles to a healthy digestion, and begin adding in those building blocks that you are lacking. If you still need more guidance, I highly recommend that you find a licensed naturopathic physician in your area. If you visit my website at www.drlaurendeville.com/gut, you will find a list of naturopathic physicians in your area.

Here's to your health, and God bless you!

Dr Lauren
www.drlaurendeville.com

Appendix A

ALLERGY ELIMINATION DIET

This protocol will help you to identify your biggest allergy triggers without IgG testing. I'd still prefer IgG testing, since that will catch even unusual allergens, but if you don't have the opportunity to do so, this will still work!

You will avoid all the foods on the "avoid" list for two weeks. After that, reintroduce a pure source of each food every three days, keeping a diet diary the whole time (see an example at the end of Appendix A) to see how you react. When you reintroduce a food, you want to add a LOT of it, so that if you react, we can tell.

FOODS TO AVOID

Dairy – including milk, cheese, butter, yogurt, sour cream, cottage cheese, whey, casein, sodium caseinate, calcium caseinate, etc.

Eggs – you must avoid not only whole eggs, but eggs included as an ingredient.

Wheat – including most breads, pasta, baked goods, flour, etc.

Corn – including any product with corn oil, vegetable oil (if not identified), corn syrup or HFCS, corn chips, corn tortillas, etc.

Soy – Soy milk, soy cheese, soy yogurt, tofu, miso soup, tofu burgers, etc.

Nightshades – avoid potatoes, eggplant, peppers, and tomatoes.

Citrus – oranges, grapefruits, lemons, limes, tangerines, etc.

Nuts – avoid peanuts and almonds. Other nuts are okay.

Refined sugars – Avoid anything ending in -ose (sucrose, glucose, dextrose, fructose), etc.

Food additives – avoid all artificial colors, flavors, preservatives, artificial sweeteners, etc.

Known allergens – avoid any food you know you are allergic to, even if it's otherwise allowed on this diet.

FOODS YOU CAN EAT

Grain and Flour – Anything 100% whole grain, as long as it is gluten free, including rice, buckwheat, potato, bean flours, millet, oats. barley, spelt (if it specifies gluten free), amaranth, and quinoa.

Legumes – Includes lentils, peas, chickpeas, navy beans, kidney beans, black beans, string beans, and others. Any dried beans should be soaked overnight, and rinsed before cooking. Canned beans aren't great for you but they will work for these purposes, provided there are no added sugars.

Vegetables – Eat lots of these; all except the nightshades and corn.

Proteins – All fish, seafood, chicken, beef, and pork are allowed.

Nuts and seeds – All nuts are allowed except for peanuts and almonds (the most common allergens). Make sure you choose those that are not sweetened; nut butters often are.

Oils and fats – choose coconut oil, grape seed oil, avocado oil, or olive oil. Avoid canola, rapeseed, and corn oils, or any unspecified vegetable oils.

Beverages – No added sugars; you can do herbal teas, coffee (though no more than one cup daily), green or black tea, seltzer water, fruit juices, coconut water, or milk substitutes (rice, hemp, flax, coconut)

Thickeners – xanthan gum, arrowroot, agar.

RETESTING INSTRUCTIONS

After two weeks, you're unlikely to feel dramatically different—but if you have food allergies and they are some of the common ones, you will likely have improved enough that when you test foods, you will still notice the difference.

Test pure sources of foods: Make sure you're testing a pure source of each food, and ideally an organic version, so that you don't get contaminants from hormones, pesticides, etc.

Test one new food every three days. The IgG immunoglobulin can have reactions that are delayed up to 72 hours.

Eat a lot of each test food. If you react, we want to know. Eat the food group at breakfast, lunch, and dinner on the first day only, and then take it back out and wait three days, while recording your symptoms in a diet diary.

Do not test foods you know are a problem for you.

Dairy test – Separate dairy by category: test milk one day, cheese another day, and yogurt another day. You may even want to separate different types of cheeses, since some people have issues with one and not another. Also consider testing goat milk or sheep milk separately, if you drink those.

Wheat test – try a pure wheat source, such as Cream of Wheat.

Corn test – try corn on the cob, ideally fresh and organic.

Egg test – Test egg whites and egg yolks separately, since some people are sensitive to one and not another. Hard boiled eggs are best for this, so that they can be easily separated.

Soy test – Test tofu or edamame.

Citrus test – Test different citrus fruits on different days.

Sugar test – test pure sugar mixed with a food you can otherwise tolerate.

Food additive test – You can purchase food dye sets and test each individual color if you wish, although I would encourage leaving these out of your diet.

Symptoms To Watch For While Adding Foods Back

General: Fatigue, anxiety, depression, insomnia, food cravings, weight gain

Infection: feeling like you're getting sick (sore throat, chills, etc)

Ear, Nose & Throat: nasal congestion, postnasal drip

Respiratory: asthma or chest tightness, difficulty breathing

Gastrointestinal: constipation, diarrhea, bloating, abdominal cramping, gallbladder pain

Cardiovascular: High blood pressure, arrhythmia, chest pain

Dermatological: Acne, eczema, psoriasis, canker sores, hives

Rheumatological: Muscle aches, joint pain

Neurological: Migraines and other headaches, numbness

Other: frequent urination, teeth grinding, bedwetting

Once Your Testing Is Completed

When you have identified the culprits, avoid them completely for six weeks, while taking nutrients to heal up your gut lining (see the end of Chapter 4). After that, you can likely reintroduce the foods in one of two ways: you may eat small amounts of the food each day, or large amounts one day, but then you cannot have that food again for three days after that. This is called a rotation diet, and will help you to avoid re-sensitization.

Diet Diary

BMs = Bowel Movements. The time is often all that's necessary, unless there's something unusual about it, in which case you should record it. Otherwise, any symptoms that come up should be recorded that show up in the above list. Continue this practice until you have reintroduced all foods into your diet that you intend to test.

	Breakfast	Lunch	Dinner	Symptoms and BMs
Day 1				
Day 2				
Day 3				
Day 4				
Day 5				
Day 6				
Day 7				

BIBLIOGRAPHY

Chapter 1

1. Tripathi, A. et al. "Identification of human zonulin, a physiological modulator of tight junctions, as prehaptoglobin-2." Proceedings of the National Academy of Sciences of the United States of America. U.S. National Library of Medicine, 15 Sept. 2009. Web. 04 Jan. 2017.

2. Duerksen, DR. "A comparison of antibody testing, permeability testing, and zonulin levels with small-bowel biopsy in celiac disease patients on a gluten-free diet." Digestive diseases and sciences. U.S. National Library of Medicine, 28 Apr. 2009. Web. 04 Jan. 2017.

3. Vanuytsel, T., S. Vermeire, and I. Cleynen. "The role of Haptoglobin and its related protein, Zonulin, in inflammatory bowel disease." Tissue barriers. U.S. National Library of Medicine, 10 Dec. 2013. Web. 04 Jan. 2017. <https://www.ncbi.nlm.nih.gov/pubmed/24868498>.

4. "Wheat: Background." *USDA ERS - Background*. N.p., 23 Nov. 2016. Web. 06 Feb. 2017. <https://www.ers.usda.gov/topics/crops/wheat/background.aspx>. Samsel, Anthony, and Stephanie Seneff.

5. Mesnage, R., N. Defarge, J. Spiroux De Vendômois, and GE Séralini. "Potential Toxic Effects of Glyphosate and Its Commercial Formulations below Regulatory Limits." National Center for Biotechnology Information. U.S. National Library of Medicine, 12 Aug. 2015. Web. 27 Sept. 2015. <http://www.ncbi.nlm.nih.gov/pubmed/26282372>.

6. Potera, Carol. "DIET AND NUTRITION: The Artificial Food Dye Blues." Environmental Health Perspectives. National Institute of Environmental Health Sciences, 1 Oct. 2010. Web. 26 Sept. 2015. <http://www.ncbi.nlm.nih.gov/pmc/articles/PMC2957945/>.

7. Hengel, M., and T. Shibamoto. "Carcinogenic 4(5)-methylimidazole Found in Beverages, Sauces, and Caramel Colors: Chemical Properties, Analysis, and Biological Activities." National Center for Biotechnology Information. U.S. National Library of Medicine, 15 Jan. 2013. Web. 26 Sept. 2015. <http://www.ncbi.nlm.nih.gov/pubmed/23294412>.

8. Beaulieu, Robert, Ronald Warwar, and Bruce Buerk. "Canthaxanthin Retinopathy with Visual Loss: A Case Report and Review." Case Reports in Ophthalmological Medicine. Hindawi Publishing Corporation, 30 Oct. 2013. Web. 26 Sept. 2015. <http://www.ncbi.nlm.nih.gov/pmc/articles/PMC3833018/>.

9. Souza, Russell, Andrew Mente, Adriana Maroleanu, Adrian Cozma, Vanessa Ha, Teruko Kishibe, Elizabeth Uleryk, Patrick Budylowski, Holger Schünemann, Joseph Beyene, and Sonia Anand. "Intake of Saturated and Trans Unsaturated Fatty Acids and Risk of All Cause Mortality, Cardiovascular Disease, and Type 2 Diabetes: Systematic Review and Meta-analysis of Observational Studies." BMJ : British Medical Journal. BMJ Publishing Group Ltd., 12 Aug. 2015. Web. 26 Sept. 2015.

10. "World Cancer Research Fund Officially Recommends Avoiding Processed Meat." CNN IReport. 22 May 2013. Web. 26 Sept. 2015. <http://ireport.cnn.com/docs/DOC-1048224>.

11. Nöthlings, U., LR Wilkens, SP Murphy, JH Hankin, BE Henderson, and LN Kolonel. "Meat and Fat Intake as Risk Factors for Pancreatic Cancer: The Multiethnic Cohort Study." National Center for Biotechnology

Information. U.S. National Library of Medicine, 5 Oct. 2005. Web. 26 Sept. 2015. <http://www.ncbi.nlm.nih.gov/pubmed/16204695>.

12. "Lower Your Cancer Risk by Eating Right." Lower Your Cancer Risk by Eating Right. American Cancer Society. Web. 26 Sept. 2015. <http://www.cancer.org/myacs/newengland/lower-your-cancer-risk-by-eating-right>.

13. Ashok, Iyaswamy, and Rathinasamy Sheeladevi. "Biochemical Responses and Mitochondrial Mediated Activation of Apoptosis on Long-term Effect of Aspartame in Rat Brain." Redox Biology. Elsevier, 29 Apr. 2014. Web. 26 Sept. 2015. <http://www.ncbi.nlm.nih.gov/pmc/articles/PMC4085354/>.

14. Zeevi, David et al. "Personalized Nutrition by Prediction of Glycemic Responses." Cell. N.p., 19 Nov. 2015. Web. 26 Dec. 2016.

15. Fowler, Sharon P.G., Ken Williams, and Helen P. Hazuda. "Diet Soda Intake Is Associated with Long-Term Increases in Waist Circumference in a Biethnic Cohort of Older Adults: The San Antonio Longitudinal Study of Aging." Wiley Online Library. Journal of the American Geriatrics Society, 17 Mar. 2015. Web. 20 Feb. 2017. <http://onlinelibrary.wiley.com/doi/10.1111/jgs.13376/abstract>.

16. Meister, B et al. "Neurotransmitters, neuropeptides and binding sites in the rat mediobasal hypothalamus: effects of monosodium glutamate (MSG) lesions." SpringerLink. Experimental Brain Research, 16 Mar. 1989. Web. 26 Dec. 2016. <http://link.springer.com/article/10.1007/BF00247894>.

17. Patterson Neubert, Amy. "Study: Trying to lose weight? Lose the fat substitutes." Pudue University News Service. Purdue University, 21 June 2011. Web. 26 Dec. 2016. <http://www.purdue.edu/newsroom/research/2011/110621SwithersObesity.html>.

18. Kurokawa, Y et al. "Toxicity and Carcinogenicity of Potassium Bromate--a New Renal Carcinogen." Environmental Health Perspectives 87 (1990): 309–335. Print.

19. Addicott, Merideth, Lucie Yang, Ann Peiffer, Luke Burnett, Jonathan Burdette, Michael Chen, Satoru Hayasaka, Robert Kraft, Joseph Maldjian, and Paul Laurienti. "The Effect of Daily Caffeine Use on Cerebral Blood Flow: How Much Caffeine Can We Tolerate?" Human Brain Mapping.

U.S. National Library of Medicine, 30 Oct. 2009. Web. 26 Sept. 2015. <http://www.ncbi.nlm.nih.gov/pmc/articles/PMC2748160/>.

20. Rizzello, Carlo G et al. "Highly Efficient Gluten Degradation by Lactobacilli and Fungal Proteases during Food Processing: New Perspectives for Celiac Disease." Applied and Environmental Microbiology 73 (2007): 4499-4507.

21. Eker, S et al. "Foliar-applied glyphosate substantially reduced uptake and transport of iron and manganese in sunflower (Helianthus annuus L.) plants." J Agric Food Chem. 2006 Dec 27; 54(26):10019-25.

22. Nachman, Keeve E et al. "Poultry Drug Increases Levels of Toxic Arsenic in Chicken Meat." Johns Hopkins, 11 May, 2013. Web 28 May 2017. <http://www.jhsph.edu/news/news-releases/2013/nachman_arsenic_chicken.html>

Chapter 2

1. Grün, Felix et al. "Endocrine-Disrupting Organotin Compounds Are Potent Inducers of Adipogenesis in Vertebrates." Endocrine-Disrupting Organotin Compounds Are Potent Inducers of Adipogenesis in Vertebrates: Molecular Endocrinology: Vol 20, No 9. Molecular Endocrinology, 07 Jan. 2009. Web. 04 Jan. 2017. <http://press.endocrine.org/doi/10.1210/me.2005-0367?url_ver=Z39.88-2003&rfr_id=ori%3Arid%3Acrossref.org&rfr_dat=cr_pub%3Dpubmed&>

2. Goodman, Michael, Judy S. LaKind, and Donald R. Mattison. " CrossRef citations 21 Altmetric Review Article Do phthalates act as obesogens in humans? A systematic review of the epidemiological literature." Taylor & Francis Online. Taylor & Francis Group, 14 Jan. 2014. Web. 04 Jan. 2017.

3. Sargis, Robert M. et al. "Environmental Endocrine Disruptors Promote Adipogenesis in the 3T3-L1 Cell Line through Glucocorticoid Receptor Activation." Obesity (Silver Spring, Md.) 18.7 (2010): 1283–1288. PMC. Web. 4 Jan. 2017.

4. Sargis, Robert M., Et al. "The novel endocrine disruptor tolylfluanid impairs insulin signaling in primary rodent and human adipocytes through a reduction in insulin receptor substrate-1 levels." Science Direct. Elsevier

B.V., 10 Oct. 2016. Web. 04 Jan. 2017. <http://www.sciencedirect.com/science/article/pii/S0925443912000439>.

5. Trasnd, Leonardo, M.D. et al. "Association Between Urinary Bisphenol A Concentration and Obesity Prevalence in Children and Adolescents." The JAMA Network. American Medical Association, 19 Sept. 2012. Web. 04 Jan. 2017. <http://jamanetwork.com/journals/jama/fullarticle/1360865>.

6. Grens, Kerry. "Obesogens." The Scientist. LabX Media Group, 1 Nov. 2015. Web. 4 Jan. 2017.

7. Tomljenovic, L., and CA Shaw. "Do Aluminum Vaccine Adjuvants Contribute to the Rising Prevalence of Autism?" National Center for Biotechnology Information. U.S. National Library of Medicine, 23 Aug. 2011. Web. 22 Oct. 2015.

8. U.S. Food and Drug Administration. "Draft Assessment of Bisphenol A for Use in Food Contact Applications," 14 August 2008. Web 29 May 2016. <https://www.fda.gov/ohrms/dockets/AC/08/briefing/2008-0038b1_01_02_FDA%20BPA%20Draft%20Assessment.pdf>

9. Krishnan, A. V. et al. "Bisphenol-A: an estrogenic substance is released from polycarbonate flasks during autoclaving." Endocrinology (1993) 132 (6): 2279-2286.

10. Bittner, George et al. "Chemicals having estrogenic activity can be released from some bisphenol a-free, hard and clear, thermoplastic resins." Environ Health. 2014; 13: 103.

11. Naish, John. "Why air fresheners and scented candles can wreck your health: They could cause cancerous DNA mutations and asthma." The Daily Mail, 2 September 2015. Web 29 May 2016. <http://www.dailymail.co.uk/femail/article-3220306/Why-air-fresheners-scented-candles-wreck-health-cause-cancerous-DNA-mutations-asthma.html>

Chapter 3

1. Shoemaker, R. *Surviving Mold.* Web. 03 Feb. 2017. <http://www.survivingmold.com/>.

2. Shoemaker, R. C., D. House, and J. C. Ryan. "Structural brain abnormalities in patients with inflammatory illness acquired following

exposure to water-damaged buildings: a volumetric MRI study using NeuroQuant®." *Neurotoxicology and teratology.* U.S. National Library of Medicine, 17 June 2014. Web. 03 Feb. 2017. <https://www.ncbi.nlm.nih.gov/pubmed/24946038

3. "Post-Treatment Lyme Disease Syndrome." *Centers for Disease Control and Prevention.* Centers for Disease Control and Prevention, 03 Nov. 2016. Web. 03 Feb. 2017. <https://www.cdc.gov/lyme/postlds/>.

4. Shoemaker, R. C., and D. E. House. "Sick building syndrome (SBS) and exposure to water-damaged buildings: time series study, clinical trial and mechanisms." *Neurotoxicology and teratology.* U.S. National Library of Medicine, 7 Aug. 2006. Web. 03 Feb. 2017. <https://www.ncbi.nlm.nih.gov/pubmed/17010568>.

Chapter 4

1. https://www.ncbi.nlm.nih.gov/pmc/articles/PMC371506/pdf/jcinvest00691-0075.pdf?_ga=1.186931240.1474313323.1478370897

2. Campbell, T. Colin, and Thomas M. Campbell. The China Study: The Most Comprehensive Study of Nutrition Ever Conducted and the Startling Implications for Diet, Weight Loss and Long-term Health. Dallas, Tex.: BenBella, 2005. Print.

3. Price, Weston A. Nutrition and Physical Degeneration. 8th ed. Lemon Grove, CA: Price-Pottenger Nutrition Foundation, 2008. Print.

4. Gordon, Serena. "Link Between Diabetes, Alzheimer's Disease Strengthened." Consumer HealthDay. HealthDay, 25 Aug. 2010. Web. 26 Sept. 2015. <http://consumer.healthday.com/cognitive-and-neurological-health-information-26/alzheimer-s-news-20/link-between-diabetes-alzheimer-s-disease-strengthened-642482.html>.

5. Paddock, Catharine. "Chocolate Gorging Linked To Opium Chemical In Brain." Medical News Today. MediLexicon International, 21 Sept. 2012. Web. 26 Sept. 2015. <http://www.medicalnewstoday.com/articles/250517.php>.

6. Kobylewski, Sarah. "CSPI Says Food Dyes Pose Rainbow of Risks ~ Newsroom ~ News from CSPI ~ Center for Science in the Public Interest."

CSPI Says Food Dyes Pose Rainbow of Risks – Newsroom – News from CSPI – Center for Science in the Public Interest. Center For Science In The Public Interest, 29 June 2010. Web. 26 Sept. 2015. <http://www.cspinet.org/new/201006291.html>.

7. Fung, Teresa, Meredith Arasaratnam, Francine Grodstein, Jeffrey Katz, Bernard Rosner, Walter Willett, and Diane Feskanich. "Soda Consumption and Risk of Hip Fractures in Postmenopausal Women in the Nurses' Health Study." The American Journal of Clinical Nutrition. American Society for Nutrition, 6 Aug. 2014. Web. 26 Sept. 2015. <http://www.ncbi.nlm.nih.gov/pmc/articles/PMC4135502/>.

8. Elliott, Sharon S., Nancy L. Keim, Judith S. Stern, Karen Teff, and Peter J. Havel. "Fructose, Weight Gain, and the Insulin Resistance Syndrome." The American Journal of Clinical Nutrition. American Society for Nutrition, 01 Nov. 2002. Web. 04 Jan. 2017. <http://ajcn.nutrition.org/content/76/5/911.full>.

9. "Yasmin Side Effects in Detail." Drugs.com. Drugs.com. Web. 22 Oct. 2015.

10. Brazier, Yvette. "One course of antibiotics disrupts gut microbiome for a year." Medical News Today. MediLexicon International, 10 Nov. 2015. Web. 04 Jan. 2017. <http://www.medicalnewstoday.com/articles/302179.php>.

11. Edgar, Julie. "Antibiotic Resistance: Expert Q&A With the CDC." WebMD. WebMD, n.d. Web. 04 Jan. 2017. <http://www.webmd.com/cold-and-flu/features/antibiotic-resistance-expert-q-a-cdc>.

12. Chedid, Victor et al. "Herbal Therapy Is Equivalent to Rifaximin for the Treatment of Small Intestinal Bacterial Overgrowth." Glob Adv Health Med. 2014 May; 3(3): 16–24.

Chapter 6

1. Colquhoun, J. "New Evidence on Fluoridation." National Center for Biotechnology Information. U.S. National Library of Medicine, 1984. Web. 27 Oct. 2015.

2. Pavelka, S., A. Babický, M. Vobecký, and J. Lener. "Effect of High Bromide Levels in the Organism on the Biological Half-life of Iodine in the Rat." National Center for Biotechnology Information. U.S. National Library of Medicine, 2001. Web. 27 Oct. 2015.

3. Van Leeuwen, FX, and B. Sangster. "The Toxicology of Bromide Ion." National Center for Biotechnology Information. U.S. National Library of Medicine, 1987. Web. 27 Oct. 2015.

4. Ain, KB, Y. Mori, and S. Refetoff. "Reduced Clearance Rate of Thyroxine-binding Globulin (TBG) with Increased Sialylation: A Mechanism for Estrogen-induced Elevation of Serum TBG Concentration." National Center for Biotechnology Information. U.S. National Library of Medicine, 1 Oct. 1987. Web. 27 Oct. 2015.

5. Gerli, S., E. Papaleo, A. Ferrari, and GC Di Renzo. "Randomized, Double Blind Placebo-controlled Trial: Effects of Myo-inositol on Ovarian Function and Metabolic Factors in Women with PCOS." National Center for Biotechnology Information. U.S. National Library of Medicine, 1 Sept. 2007. Web. 27 Oct. 2015.

6. Costantino, D., G. Minozzi, F. Minozzi, and C. Guaraldi. "Metabolic and Hormonal Effects of Myo-inositol in Women with Polycystic Ovary Syndrome: A Double-blind Trial." Eur Rev Med Pharmacol Sci 13.N. 2: 105-10. Print.

7. Raffone, E., P. Rizzo, and V. Benedetto. "Insulin Sensitiser Agents Alone and in Co-treatment with R-FSH for Ovulation Induction in PCOS Women." National Center for Biotechnology Information. U.S. National Library of Medicine, 26 Apr. 2010. Web. 27 Oct. 2015.

8. Muraleedharan, Vakkat, and T. Hugh Jones. "Testosterone and the Metabolic Syndrome." *Therapeutic Advances in Endocrinology and Metabolism*. SAGE Publications, Oct. 2010. Web. 11 July 2017.

9. Kadi, F. "Cellular and Molecular Mechanisms Responsible for the Action of Testosterone on Human Skeletal Muscle. A Basis for Illegal Performance Enhancement." *British Journal of Pharmacology*. Nature Publishing Group, June 2008. Web. 11 July 2017.

10. Goglia, L., V. Tosi, A.M. Sanchez, M.I. Flamini, X.-D. Fu, S. Zullino, A.R. Genazzani, and T. Simoncini. "Endothelial Regulation of ENOS, PAI-1 and T-PA by Testosterone and Dihydrotestosterone in Vitro and in Vivo." *MHR: Basic Science of Reproductive Medicine.* Oxford University Press, 14 June 2010. Web. 11 July 2017.

11. Iranmanesh, Ali, Donna Lawson, and Johannes D. Veldhuis. "Glucose Ingestion Acutely Lowers Pulsatile LH and Basal Testosterone Secretion in Men." *American Journal of Physiology - Endocrinology and Metabolism.* American Physiological Society, 15 Mar. 2012. Web. 11 July 2017.

12. Traish, A. M., A. Haider, G. Doros, and F. Saad. "Long-term Testosterone Therapy in Hypogonadal Men Ameliorates Elements of the Metabolic Syndrome: An Observational, Long-term Registry Study." *International Journal of Clinical Practice.* N.p., 15 Oct. 2013. Web. 11 July 2017.

13. "Generational Decline in Testosterone Levels Observed." Healio. Endocrine Today, 1 Feb. 2007. Web. 27 Oct. 2015.

14. Patterson, TR, JD Stringham, and AW Meikle. "Nicotine and Cotinine Inhibit Steroidogenesis in Mouse Leydig Cells." National Center for Biotechnology Information. U.S. National Library of Medicine, 1990. Web. 27 Oct. 2015.

15. Lucero, J., BL Harlow, RL Barbieri, P. Sluss, and DW Cramer. "Early Follicular Phase Hormone Levels in Relation to Patterns of Alcohol, Tobacco, and Coffee Use." National Center for Biotechnology Information. U.S. National Library of Medicine, 1 Oct. 2001. Web. 27 Oct. 2015.

16. Ferrini, Rebecca L., and Elizabeth Barrett-Connor. "Caffeine Intake and Endogenous Sex Steroid Levels in Postmenopausal Women." American Journal of Epidemiology (1996): 642-44. Print.

Chapter 8

1. Obregon-Tito et al. (2015). Subsistence strategies in traditional societies distinguish gut microbiomes. *Nat Commun* 6, 6505. Doi: 10. 1038/ ncomms7505.

2. Schnorr et al. (2014). Gut microbiome of the Hadza hunter-gatherers. *Nat Commun*, 5, 3654. doi: 10. 1038/ncomms4654.

3. De Fillippo et al. (2010). Impact of diets in shaping gut microbiota revealed by a comparative study in children form Europe and rural Africa. *Proc Natl Acad Sci U S A*, 107(33), 14691-14696.

Chapter 9

1. Graham, Drew. "How Vegetable Oils Replaced Animal Fats in the American Diet." The Atlantic. Atlantic Media Company, 26 Apr. 2012. Web. 13 Nov. 2015. <http://www.theatlantic.com/health/archive/2012/04/how-vegetable-oils-replaced-animal-fats-in-the-american-diet/256155/>.

2. Campbell, T. Colin. The China Study: The Most Comprehensive Study of Nurtrition Ever Conducted and the Startling Implications for Diet, Weight Loss and Long-term Health. Dallas, TX.: Banbella, 2006. Print.

3. Landers, Timothy, Bevin Cohen, Thomas Wittum, and Elaine Larson. "A Review of Antibiotic Use in Food Animals: Perspective, Policy, and Potential." Public Health Reports. Association of Schools of Public Health, 2012. Web. 13 Nov. 2015. <http://www.ncbi.nlm.nih.gov/pmc/articles/PMC3234384/>.

4. "Nutrition-Related Issues." FAO. Agriculture and Consumer Protection. Web. 13 Nov. 2015. <http://www.fao.org/wairdocs/ae584e/ae584e05.htm>.

5. Walton, Alice G. "How Much Sugar Are Americans Eating?" Forbes. Forbes Magazine, 30 Aug. 2012. Web. 13 Nov. 2015. <http://www.forbes.com/sites/alicegwalton/2012/08/30/how-much-sugar-are-americans-eating-infographic/>.

Chapter 10

1. Washington State University. "Commercial organic farms have better fruit and soil, lower environmental impact, study finds." ScienceDaily. ScienceDaily, 2 September 2010. <www.sciencedaily.com/releases/2010/09/100901171553.htm>.

Chapter 11

1. Lappe, Joan M, Diane Travers-Gustafson, K Michael Davies, Robert R Recker, and Robert P Heaney. "Vitamin D and Calcium Supplementation Reduces Cancer Risk: Results of a Randomized Trial." The American Journal of Clinical Nutrition 85.6 (2007): 1586-591. Print.

2. Mead, M. "Benefits of Sunlight: A Bright Spot for Human Health." Environmental Health Perspectives. National Institute of Environmental Health Sciences, 1 Apr. 2008. Web. 13 Nov. 2015. <http://www.ncbi.nlm. nih.gov/pmc/articles/PMC2290997/>.

3. "Vitamin D Deficiency Linked More Closely to Diabetes than Obesity." Vitamin D Deficiency Linked More Closely to Diabetes than Obesity. Endocrine Society, 23 Feb. 2015. Web. 13 Nov. 2015. <https://www. endocrine.org/news-room/current-press-releases/vitamin-d-deficiency-linked-more-closely-to-diabetes-than-obesity>.

4. Munger, K. L., S. M. Zhang, E. O'reilly, M. A. Hernan, M. J. Olek, W. C. Willett, and A. Ascherio. "Vitamin D Intake and Incidence of Multiple Sclerosis." Neurology 62.1 (2004): 60-65. Penn State. American Academy of Neurology. Web. 13 Nov. 2015.

5. Pearson, Catherine. "Can Vitamin D Help With Cramps?" The Huffington Post. TheHuffingtonPost.com, 27 Feb. 2012. Web. 13 Nov. 2015. <http:// www.huffingtonpost.com/2012/02/27/vitamin-d-pms-menstrual-cramps-italy_n_1305127.html>.

6. Grogan, Martha. "Calcium Supplements: A Risk Factor for Heart Attack?" *Mayo Clinic.* Mayo Foundation for Medicl Education and Research, 19 Apr. 2013. Web. 15 Nov. 2015. <http://www.mayoclinic.org/diseases-conditions/heart-attack/expert-answers/calcium-supplements/faq-20058352>

7. "Calcium beyond the Bones - Harvard Health." *Harvard Health.* Harvard Health Publications, 1 Mar. 2010. Web. 15 Nov. 2015. <http://www. health.harvard.edu/womens-health/calcium-beyond-the-bones>

8. Paddock, Catharine. "Sun Exposure Benefits May Outweigh Risks Say Scientists." Medical News Today. MediLexicon International, 8 May 2013. Web. 13 Nov. 2015. <http://www.medicalnewstoday.com/articles/260247. php>.

9. Mead, M. "Benefits of Sunlight: A Bright Spot for Human Health." Environmental Health Perspectives. National Institute of Environmental Health Sciences, 1 Apr. 2008. Web. 13 Nov. 2015. <http://www.ncbi.nlm. nih.gov/pmc/articles/PMC2290997/>.

Chapter 12

1. "Insufficient Sleep Is a Public Health Problem." Centers for Disease Control and Prevention. U.S. Department of Health and Human Services, 3 Sept. 2015. Web. 13 Nov. 2015. <http://www.cdc.gov/features/dssleep/>.
2. Meco, Antonio Di, Yash B. Joshi, and Domenico Praticò. "Sleep Deprivation Impairs Memory, Tau Metabolism, and Synaptic Integrity of a Mouse Model of Alzheimer's Disease with Plaques and Tangles." Neurobiology of Aging 35.8 (2014): 1813-820. Neurobiology of Aging. Elsevier. Web. 13 Nov. 2015.
3. Kawai, N., N. Sakai, M. Okuro, S. Karakawa, Y. Tsuneyoshi, N. Kawasaki, T. Takeda, M. Bannai, and S. Nishino. "The Sleep-promoting and Hypothermic Effects of Glycine Are Mediated by NMDA Receptors in the Suprachiasmatic Nucleus." National Center for Biotechnology Information. U.S. National Library of Medicine, 23 Dec. 2014. Web. 13 Nov. 2015. <http://www.ncbi.nlm.nih.gov/pubmed/25533534>.

Chapter 14

1. Covey, Stephen R. The 7 Habits of Highly Effective People: Powerful Lessons in Personal Change. 25th Anniversary ed. Simon & Schuster, 2013. Print.
2. Wenner, Melinda. "Smile! It Could Make You Happier." Scientific American Global RSS. Scientific American, 1 Aug. 2009. Web. 23 Sept. 2015. <http://www.scientificamerican.com/article/smile-it-could-make-you-happier>.
3. Martin, Hugo. "More than Half of Americans Have Gone 12 Months without a Vacation." Los Angeles Times. Los Angeles Times, 13 Aug. 2015. Web. 23 Sept. 2015. <http://www.latimes.com/business/la-fi-12-months-without-a-vacation-20150813-story.html>.
4. Renzulli, Kerri Anne. "How to Disconnect from Work This Vacation." Time. Time, 18 July 2014. Web. 23 Sept. 2015. <http://time.com/

money/2982053/unplug-disconnect-work-vacation-career-boss-email-
phone/>.

5. Eaker, Elaine D., Joan Pinsky, and William P. Castelli. "Myocardial
   Infarction and Coronary Death among Women: Psychosocial Predictors
   from a 20-Year Follow-up of Women in the Framingham Study." American
   Journal of Epidemiology 135.8 (1992): 854-64. Oxford Journals. Oxford
   University Press. Web. 23 Sept. 2015. <http://aje.oxfordjournals.org/
   content/135/8/854.short>.

6. Virtanen, Marianna, Katriina Heikkilä, Markus Jokela, Jane E. Ferrie, G.
   David Batty, Jussi Vahtera, and Mika Kivimäki. "Long Working Hours
   and Coronary Heart Disease: A Systematic Review and Meta-Analysis."
   American Journal of Epidemiology 176.7 (2012): 586-96. Oxford Journals.
   Oxford University Press. Web. 23 Sept. 2015. <http://aje.oxfordjournals.
   org/content/176/7/586>.

7. Virtanen M, Stansfeld SA, Fuhrer R, Ferrie JE, Kivimäki M (2012)
   Overtime Work as a Predictor of Major Depressive Episode: A 5-Year
   Follow-Up of the Whitehall II Study. PLoS ONE 7(1): e30719.
   doi:10.1371/journal.pone.0030719 Web. 23 Sept. 2015. <http://journals.
   plos.org/plosone/article?id=10.1371/journal.pone.0030719>

8. Virtanen, Marianna, Archana Singh-Manoux, Jane E. Ferrie, David
   Gimeno, Michael G. Marmot, Marko Elovainio, Markus Jokela, Jussi
   Vahtera, and Mika Kivimäki. "Long Working Hours and Cognitive
   Function The Whitehall II Study." American Journal of Epidemiology
   169.5 (2009): 596-605. Oxford Journals. Oxford University Press. Web.
   23 Sept. 2015. <10.1093/aje/kwn382>.

9. Fritz, Charlotte, and Sabine Sonnentag. "Recovery, Well-being, and
   Performance-related Outcomes: The Role of Workload and Vacation
   Experiences." Journal of Applied Psychology 91.4 (2006): 936-45. APA
   PsycNET. American Psychological Association. Web. 23 Sept. 2015.
   <http://psycnet.apa.org/journals/apl/91/4/936/>.

10. Casey, John. "Do You Know How Much Sugar You're Eating?"
    MedicineNet. MedicineNet, 16 Dec. 2003. Web. 21 Nov. 2015. <http://
    www.medicinenet.com/script/main/art.asp?articlekey=56589>.

Chapter 15

1. Cloud, Henry, and John Sims Townsend. Boundaries: When to Say Yes, How to Say No, to Take Control of Your Life. Zondervan, 1992. Print.

2. Boyles, Salynn. "Happiness Is Contagious." WebMD. WebMD, 4 Dec. 2008. Web. 23 Sept. 2015.

3. Gladwell, Malcolm. Outliers: The Story of Success. Little, Brown, 2008. Print.

4. Chapter 16

5. Maslow, Abraham H. A Theory of Human Motivation. Martino Fine, 2013. Print.

6. Ferriss, Timothy. The 4-hour Workweek: Escape 9-5, Live Anywhere, and Join the New Rich. Expanded and Updated Ed., 1st Revised ed. New York: Crown, 2009. Print.

7. Seligman, Martin E. P. Learned Optimism: How to Change Your Mind and Your Life. New York: Vintage, 2006. Print.

8. Frankl, Viktor E. Man's Search for Meaning. Boston: Beacon, 2006. Print.

9. Amen, Daniel G. Change Your Brain, Change Your Life: The Breakthrough Program for Conquering Anxiety, Depression, Obsessiveness, Anger, and Impulsiveness. New York: Times, 2000. Print.

10. Hruby, Patrick. "Washington Was Making Rep. Tim Ryan Sick ... until He Found Mindfulness." Washington Times. The Washington Times, 11 July 2012. Web. 25 Sept. 2015. <http://www.washingtontimes.com/news/2012/jul/11/ohio-democrat-uses-mindfulness-stress-reduction-te/?page=1>.

11. Emmons, Robert A. Thanks!: how practicing gratitude can make you happier. New York: Houghton Mifflin, 2008. Print.

12. Avvenuti, G., I. Baiardini, and A. Giardini. "Optimism's Explicative Role for Chronic Diseases." Frontiers in psychology. U.S. National Library of Medicine, 2 Mar. 2016. Web. 28 Jan. 2017. <https://www.ncbi.nlm.nih.gov/pubmed/26973582>.

13. Sirios, F. M., and A. M. Wood. "Gratitude uniquely predicts lower depression in chronic illness populations: A longitudinal study of inflammatory bowel disease and arthritis." Health psychology: official journal of the Division of Health Psychology, American Psychological Association. U.S. National Library of Medicine, 27 Oct. 2016. Web. 28 Jan. 2017.

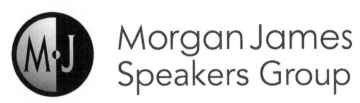

Morgan James
Speakers Group

We connect Morgan James published authors with live and online events and audiences who will benefit from their expertise.

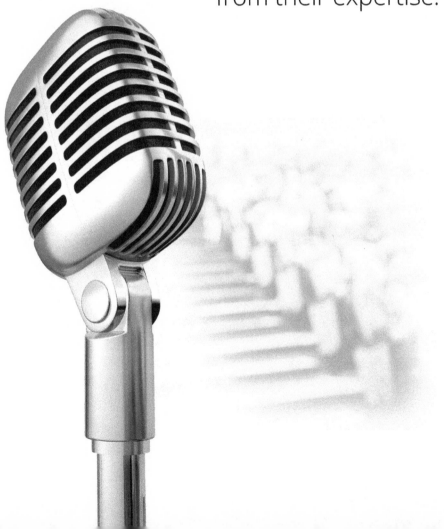

 Morgan James makes all of our titles available
through the Library for All Charity Organization.

www.LibraryForAll.org

Printed in the USA
CPSIA information can be obtained
at www.ICGtesting.com
JSHW02221514082
68134JS00018B/1059